INTRODUCTION

Step 1 of the United States Medical Licensing Examination (USMLE) is a 2-day examination in the basic medical sciences. This is a test of approximately 720 questions covering anatomy, biochemistry, microbiology, immunology, physiology, pathology, pharmacology, neurology and behavioral sciences, taken by most of the American and Canadian medical students. All candidates for the U.S. medical licensure must pass step 1, step 2 and step 3 of the USMLE in order to obtain the american medical licensure. Foreign medical graduates or physicians whose basic medical degree was conferred by a medical school located outside the United States, also must pass these examinations in order to apply for license, training or residence in the U.S.

MAURICIO LUDER M. D.
EDITOR
DIRECTOR MAVAL
MEDICAL EDUCATION
Instructor in Basic Sciences
and Clinical Sciences at
UNIVERSITY OF COLORADO

First Edition ISBN 1-884083-08-0
1997 by MAVAL Publishing, Inc. Denver, Colorado
Printed in Chile

The MAVAL MEDICAL EDUCATION board expends great efforts to make unambiguous, and medically accurate questions. However, new information may make a previously correct answer to an item incorrect, or may be a source of ambiguity not previously visualized. If inaccuracies and ambiguities occur, consult your references.

USMLE step 1

BASIC MEDICAL SCIENCES

BOOK F TEST 1

Questions: 90 Time: 90 minutes

1. Which of the following conditions does NOT favor the denaturation of a double stranded DNA molecule?

a) Incubation at 70° C
b) Incubation at low pH (pH<3).
c) Incubation with a restriction endonuclease and a single-stranded DNA-binding protein.
d) Incubation at high pH (pH>10)
e) A high G-C content

2. The first heart sound (S_1) represents:

a) the opening of the mitral and tricuspid valves
b) the closure of the mitral and tricuspid valves
c) the opening of the aortic and pulmonic valves
d) the closure of the aortic and pulmonic valves
e) the opening of the left sided heart valves

Items 3-6

Select the appropriate drug in the management of hypertension (HTN) and congestive heart failure (CHF).

a) Digoxin
b) Digitoxin
c) Captopril
d) Propranolol
e) None of the above

3. Preferred for a patient with CHF and impaired renal function.

4. It lowers peripheral vascular resistance with improvent in CHF and HTN.

5. It reduces the oxygen requirement of heart muscle, decreases the cardiac output, and protects the heart against myocardial infarction.

6. It increases the level of circulating bradykinins and decreases the sodium retention by decreasing the circulating levels of aldosterone.

7. In the middle cranial fossa, the maxillary nerve travels from the trigeminal ganglion to the pterygopalatine fossa by passing through the:

a) superior orbital fissure
c) foramen ovale
c) foramen lacerum
d) foramen spinosum
e) foramen rotundum

8. According to the Piaget theory at which of the following stages of development do school-age (7-11 years) children operate?

a) Preoperational
b) Sensorimotor
c) Formal operations
d) Autonomous operations
e) Concrete operations

9. In the Sanger or synthetic DNA sequencing procedure, the purpose of mixing dideoxynucleotides (ddNTPs) with deoxynucleotide (dNTPs) is:

a) to use ddNTPs as primers to initiate polymerization of target sequence
b) because ddNTPs are not recognized by the DNA polymerase, they are not incorporated into the growing strand
c) by incorporating ddNTPs to prevent further phosphodiester bond formation
d) by incorporating ddNTPs to alter the three-dimensional structure of the DNA molecule, which promotes denaturation under less stringent conditions
e) by incorporating ddNTPs to decrease the speed of polymerization, which allows the reaction to be stopped after a specific number of bases have been incorporated

10. On physical examination, a third year medical student notices a split S_2 (split second heart sound). What process is most likely behind this phenomenon?

a) A premature ventricular contraction
b) A prolonged interval between atrial and ventricular contraction
c) A delay between the closure of the aortic and pulmonic valves
d) Stenosis of the mitral valve
e) A bacterial vegetation on the pulmonic valve

11. The antigen binding site on an antibody is formed by the:

a) constant regions of the light chains
b) constant regions of the heavy and light chains
c) variable regions of the light chains and constant regions of the heavy chains
d) variable regions of the light and heavy chains
e) variable regions of the heavy chains and constant regions of the light chains

12. A 48 year-old woman began feeling fatigued and depressed seven months ago. In the last four weeks she has developed dementia, aphasia, rigidity, and increased deep tendon reflexes. Her family history is noncontributory. Her past medical history is remarkable for a hysterectomy 14 years ago, cholecystectomy 9 years ago, and a corneal transplant 5 years ago. What is the MOST likely diagnosis?

a) Tertiary syphilis
b) Progressive multifocal leukencephalopathy
c) Creutzfield-Jakob disease
d) Huntington's chorea
e) Alzheimer's disease

13. The following are MOST common signs and symptoms of an apical lung tumor (Pancoast's tumor), EXCEPT:

a) ptosis
b) mydriasis
c) anhydrosis
d) hemoptysis
e) dyspnea

14. The MOST likely change(s) that occur(s) during a period of stress or anxiety is:

a) an increase in lymphocyte count
b) an increase in natural killer cell reactivity
c) an increase in mitogenic response
d) an increase in stimulation of the anterior hypothalamus
e) an increase in 17-OH corticosteroids in the urine

15. A woman complains of double vision and difficulty in going down stairs. She says she tries to compensate by tilting her head to the right. On examination, she is found to have a weakness in downward gaze in the left eye while looking medially. The lesion is most likely located in the:

a) left oculomotor nerve
b) left trochlear nerve
c) left abducent nerve
d) right oculomotor nerve
e) right trochlear nerve

16. Each of the following statements regarding the natural immunity is correct, EXCEPT:

a) includes natural killer (NK) cells
b) includes interferons (IFNs)
c) includes the mucus membranes
d) involves specific recognition of antigen
e) does not require previous contact with an antigen

17. A 60-year-old white male comes to the office with bilateral paralysis of the muscles of facial expression. In this patent, the most likely level of the damage is:

a) medulla
b) pons
c) midbrain
d) diencephalon
e) cavernous sinus

18. Which of the following experimental conditions is LEAST likely to induce immunological tolerance?

a) Administering a very high dose of antigen
b) Using a dodecopeptide consisting of ten leucine-serine dimers as the antigen
c) Introducing an antigen to an adult rather than a neonatal animal
d) Administering an antigen along with cyclosporine A (CsA)
e) Administering an antigen in soluble rather than aggregated form

19. A patient who has trouble with memory consolidation most likely has a lesion of the:

a) frontal lobe
b) parietal lobe
c) hippocampus
d) hypothalamus
e) limbic lobe

20. A 17 year-old teenager is seen in the clinic for weakness. She has a history of anorexia nervosa with at least three admissions to the psychiatric unit. Regarding this condition, which of the following statements is CORRECT?

a) It is rarely fatal (less than 1% of cases)
b) It is only seen in women between age 13 and 20
c) Dieting continues despite an awareness of being too thin
d) Usually accompanied by amenorrhea
e) Etiology is mainly due to a lack of appetite

21. Compared to other polymerase enzymes, which feature of *Taq* polymerase has made it very useful in increasing the ease and efficiency of performing PCR?

a) It works optimally at higher temperatures
b) It has a more accurate proofreading activity
c) Its three-dimensional structure allows it to binds its target with greater affinity
d) Its great abundance in nature makes it relatively inexpensive to isolate and purify
e) It is highly resistant to denaturation at extremes of pH

22. Which of the following parameters is most consistently DECREASED during pregnancy?

a) Heart rate
b) Blood volume
c) Systemic vascular resistance
d) Stroke volume
e) Left ventricular end diastolic pressure

23. A 45 year-old man being treated for depression complains of feeling dizzy when he stands up. He also noticed a prolongation in his penile erections. The antidepressant that most likely is responsible for these symptoms is:

a) amitriptyline
b) trazodone
c) oxazepam
d) desipramine
e) fluoxetine

24. Which of the following statements regarding the vascularization around the spinal cord is CORRECT?

a) The anterior and posterior spinal arteries travel in the vertebral foramen.
b) The anterior spinal artery is unpaired and supplies the anterior 2/3 of the spinal cord.
c) The posterior spinal artery is unpaired and supplies the posterior 1/3 of the spinal cord.
d) The posterior spinal artery travels through the transverse foraminae of the first six cervical vertebrae
e) The posterior spinal arteries are paired and supply the posterior 2/3 of the spinal cord.

25. A Swiss psychiatrist Eugen Bleuler coined the term «schizophrenia,» and described the principal signs of this disease which called the «four A's». These «four A's» include each of the following signs, EXCEPT:

a) alienation
b) autism
c) affective blunting
d) associational loosening
e) ambivalence

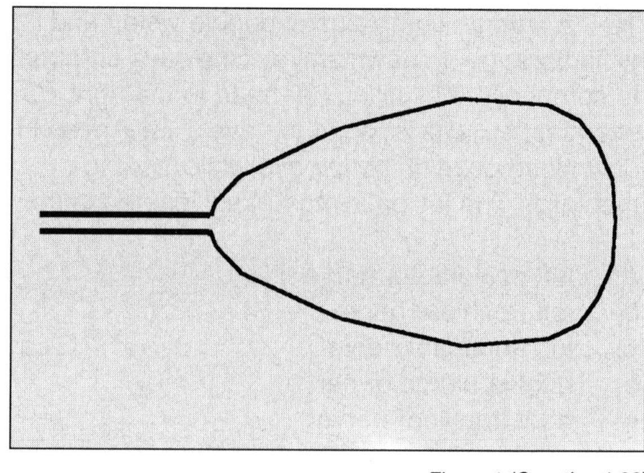

Figure 1 (Question 1.26)

26. Which of the following RNA sequences could be responsible for the stem-loop structure illustrated in figure 1?

a) 5'-gauccg —/— gauccg-3'
b) 5'-guuaau —/— aacgug-3'
c) 5'-gauccg —/— gcctag-3'
d) 5'-gauccg —/— cggauc-3'
e) 5'-gauccg —/— cuaggc-3'

27. The opiod drug methadone:

a) has an abuse potential lower than that for morphine
b) rapidly reverses an overdose of heroin because it is an opioid receptor antagonist
c) cannot be administered orally
d) is frequently used for post-operative analgesia
e) has a longer serum half-life than that of morphine

28. Which one of the following drugs can be administered causing LEAST toxicity, in a patient who has been identified as a «slow acetylator?»

a) Acetaminophen
b) Sulfadiazine
c) Isoniazid
d) Lorazepam
e) Procainamide

29. Which of the following statements regarding the methods of contraception is MOST accurate?

a) Oral contraceptives are associated with an increased risk of ovarian and endometrial cancer
b) Up to 30% of women who use transdermal progestin patches are never able to become pregnant after its removal
c) The failure rate of the condom is higher than that of the cervical cap
d) Users of condoms and diaphragms have a lower incidence of cervical cancer
e) For a monogamous couple, using spermicidal agents alone is equally effective in preventing pregnancy as using condoms alone

30. Each of the following correctly matches the members of a normal flora present at given anatomical sites, EXCEPT:

	Location	Organism
a)	nose	*Staphylococcus aureus*
b)	throat	*Viridans streptococci*
c)	urinary bladder	*Staphylococcus epidermidis*
d)	colon	*Bacteroides fragilis*
e)	vagina	*Lactobacillus*

31. According to Cloninger's biosocial hypothesis linking personality and neurotransmitters, which neurotransmitter is MOST likely associated with novelty seeking?

a) Norepinephrine
b) Cholecystokinin (CCK)
c) GABA
d) Dopamine
e) Serotonin

32. The following statements regarding the genes encoding immunoglobulins are correct, EXCEPT:

a) there is a separate set of gene segments for the light and heavy chain pools
b) the genes for kappa and lambda light chains are located on separate chromosomes
c) both light and heavy chains gene pools contain C, V, D, and J genes
d) the total number of different V gene segments outnumbers the total number of D, J and C gene segments
e) in B-lymphocytes, immunoglobulin genes (and not their gene products) are rearranged

Items 33-34

Item 33

In an experiment to restore hind limb function to rats with spinal cord transections, which of the following experimental designs to circumvent the lesion would be MOST promising?

a) Linking central nervous system (CNS) axons with peripheral nervous system (PNS) cell bodies
b) Linking PNS axons with CNS cell bodies
c) Linking CNS axons to CNS axons
d) Linking CNS cell bodies to CNS cell bodies
e) Linking PNS axons to PNS cell bodies

Item 34

In the above experiment, it is decided to stabilize the new connections and to encourage growth by equipping the axons with fibrin linked to a signaling molecule. Which signaling molecule might be most effective at stimulating nerve growth?

a) Fibroblast growth factor (FGF)
b) Epidermal growth factor (EGF)
c) Erythropoietin (EPO)
d) Interleukin 8 (IL-8)
e) Granulocyte-macrophage colony stimulating factor (GM-CSF)

51. Which of the following BEST describes the decerebrate posturing?

a) Ipsilateral flexion and contralateral extension of the limbs
b) Flexion of upper limbs and extension of lower limbs
c) Extension of upper limbs and flexion of lower limbs
d) Extension of upper and lower limbs
e) Flexion of upper and lower limbs

Items 52-54

Match the appropriate imaging technique with the descriptions below.

A) Computed tomography (CT) scan
B) Positron emission tomography (PET) scan
C) Magnetic resonance imaging (MRI)
D) Electroencephalogram (EEG)
E) X-ray with fluorescent dye

52. High spatial and contrast resolution, based upon spinning nuclei.

53. A two-dimensional view is reconstructed from multiple one-dimensional projections at different angles; limited by contrast resolution.

54. Most useful in demonstrating changes in blood flow and oxygenation that result from neuronal activity.

55. In a case of disputed paternity, the following blood types are obtained:

Ms. Y: B, Rh(D)-
Mr. X: A, Rh(D)+
Child: O, Rh(D)+

Which of the following statements is CORRECT?

a) Ms. Y could be the mother, but Mr. X cannot be the biological father of the child
b) Mr. X could be the father, but Ms. Y could not be the natural mother of the child
c) Neither Mr. X nor Ms. Y could be the child's biological parents
d) The child could be the natural offspring of Mr. X and Ms. Y
e) No conclusion may be drawn without knowing whether Ms. Y has other children

Items 56-60

Match the following drugs with its correct features.

a) Heparin
b) Warfarin
c) Ticlopidine
d) Aspirin
e) None of the above

56. It interacts with antithrombin III to prevent coagulation.

57. It blocks thromboxane A_2 synthesis from arachidonic acid in platelets.

58. Drug with an anticoagulant effect potentiated by the concomitant use of cimetidine, cotrimoxazole, or metronidazole.

59. It is produced in human mast cells.

60. It is an non-salicylate antiplatelet drug used for prophylaxis of thrombotic stroke.

61. The «anatomical snuffbox»:

a) is a depression in the maxilla
b) is formed by the tendons of the adductor pollicis, extensor carpi radialis brevis, and the extensor pollicis longus
c) is formed by the tendons of the flexor pollicis brevis, first dorsal interosseous, and opponens pollicis
d) is formed by the pisohamate ligament and the tendons of the flexor digiti minimi and opponens digiti minimi
e) is formed by the tendons of the extensor pollicis brevis, abductor pollicis longus, and extensor pollicis brevis

62. The intravenous administration of an unknown agent into a young adult resulted in an increased stroke volume, increased systolic and diastolic blood pressure, an increase in total peripheral resistance, and a decrease in heart rate. The most likely agent is:

a) epinephrine
b) dopamine
c) acetylcholine
d) norepinephrine
e) nitric oxide

63. Which of the following conditions is commonly treated with a protein generated by recombinant DNA technology?

a) Sickle-cell anemia
b) Ankylosing spondylosis
c) Osteosarcoma
d) Juvenile-onset diabetes mellitus
e) Aspergillosis

64. A 20 year-old white male complains of diarrhea for two days. You suspect that the disease process is an acute gastroenteritis and you are prescribing an anti-diarrheic medicine. Which of the following opioid drugs would be most appropriate for treating this patient?

a) Morphine
b) Meperidine
c) Proproxyphene
d) Codeine
e) Diphenoxylate

65. Which of the following is the most potent endogenous vasoconstrictor?

a) Prostacyclin
b) Angiotensin I
c) Nitric oxide
d) Heparin
e) Endothelin

66. Which of the following defense mechanisms is the LEAST adaptive or mature?

a) Sublimation
b) Altruism
c) Humor
d) Anticipation
e) Projection

67. All of the following are functions of the frontal lobes, EXCEPT:

a) concentration
b) reading comprehension
c) language
d) judgment
e) motor regulation

68. Which of the following describes an actual regulatory interaction between cytokines?

TGF = transforming growth factor
TNF = tumor necrosis factor
IFN = interferon

a) IL-4 stimulates alpha IFN production, while IL-5 limits alpha IFN production.
b) IL-6 stimulates TGFß production, while IL-9 limits TGFß production.
c) IL-2 stimulates alpha IFN production, while gamma IFN limits alpha IFN production.
d) IL-9 stimulates TNF alpha production, while IL-4 limits TNF alpha production.
e) IL-12 stimulates gamma IFN production, while IL-10 limits gamma IFN production

69. Biological effects of bacterial endotoxin include each of the following, EXCEPT:

a) paralysis due to blockage of acetylcholine release
b) fever due to release of interleukin-1
c) shock and hypotension due to bradykinin-induced vasodilation and increased vascular permeability
d) disseminated intravascular coagulation (DIC) due to activation of Hageman factor (factor XII)
e) inflammation due to activation of the alternate pathway of complement

Items 70-71

A 54 year-old white man is having difficulty recognizing the faces of his family members. He does not meet the diagnostic criteria for dementia, and has no apparent movement disorders.

70. Which of the following terms describes his inability to recognize faces?

a) Lethologica
b) Agnosia
c) Synesthesia
d) Noesis
e) Prosopagnosia

71. A medical resident orders a CT scan to explore the presumptive diagnosis of a cerebrovascular accident (CVA). In which part of the brain is MOST likely the location of a CVA in this patient?

a) Parietal lobe
b) Frontal lobe
c) Occipital lobe
d) Limbic lobe
e) Thalamus

Items 72-74

Match the human leukocyte antigen (HLA) genes with their appropriate features.

a) A locus
b) B locus
c) C locus
d) DR locus
e) Class III locus

72. This locus encodes two complement components (C2 and C4).

73. A patient presenting with arthritis, conjunctivitis, and urethritis might have a specific haplotype at this locus.

74. This locus expresses a major histocompatibility (MHC) protein which binds helper T lymphocytes.

75. The measles virus has been found to increase IL-4 production and decrease IL-2 and gamma IFN production. Which of the following is the most likely result of these effects?

a) A substantial decline in cell-mediated immunity (CMI)
b) A substantial decline in humoral immunity
c) A substantial decline in both CMI and humeral immunity
d) A hyperreactive CMI response
e) Increased production of antigen-presenting cells (APC)

76. Resistance to which of the following antibiotics is most likely to be mediated by methylation of ribosomal RNA?

a) Aminoglycosides
b) Erythromycin
c) Penicillin
d) Quinolones
e) Sulfonamides

77. It is noticed that, when interested or afraid, a cat's pupils become larger. Which system is most likely responsible for this observation?

a) Sympathetic system
b) Parasympathetic system
c) Somatic nervous system
d) Dopaminegeric system
e) Increased serotonin conductance

Items 78-79

Select the best answer from the following list.

a) Proproxyphene
b) Chloropromazine
c) Dextroamphetamine
d) Diazepam
e) Phenobarbital

78. It can paradoxically cause hyperactivity in children.

79. Used to treat attention deficit disorder with hyperactivity.

80. A 73 year-old woman in previous good health is brought to the hospital. She has been «acting strangely» for the past three days. She has seemed disoriented and has shouted unintelligibly at times. She has forgotten the name of her cat, and has been reaching out her arms as if trying to grab something unseen. She has had two episodes of urinary incontinence. Her symptoms are worse at night. During the exam, she seems perplexed, and falls asleep twice. She is febrile (101°F) and her oxygen saturation is 75%. Which diagnosis is most likely?

a) Dementia, alzheimer's type
b) Dementia, non-Alzheimer's
c) Delirium
d) Huntington's chorea
e) Pick's disease

81. A restriction endonuclease with which of the following characteristics would be especially useful in long-range physical mapping of a large genome?

a) Recognition of a specific eight-base sequence
b) Cleavage between a purine and a pyrimidine whenever such a dimer is encountered
c) Cleavage at site exactly 100 bases upstream from the recognition site
d) Stability over a narrow temperature range
e) Cleavage so as to produce only blunt ends

82. Which of the following responses most predictably follows the interaction of the mu (μ) opioid receptor with its preferred ligand?

a) Analgesia
b) Respiratory depression
c) Cognitive and behavioral disturbance
d) Hallucination
e) Cough suppression

Items 83-84

Match the following drugs used to treat peptic acid disorders with the descriptions below.

a) Calcium carbonate
b) Cimetidine
c) Misoprostol
d) Omeprazole
e) Propantheline

83. A muscarinic receptor antagonist which promotes mucosal healing by blocking the vagus nerve.

84. A prostaglandin derivative which increases mucus production but is absolutely contraindicated in pregnancy.

85. For which one of the following types of studies would relative risk be calculated?

a) Prospective
b) Retrospective
c) Cross-sectional
d) Case-control
e) Crossover

86. Selection of recombinant DNA molecules (as opposed to wild-type or nonrecombinant DNA molecules) introduced into bacteria is most readily done using which of the following techniques?

a) Estimating the length with scanning electron microscopy
b) Determining molecular weight using gel electrophoresis
c) Incubation with a radiolabelled probe specific for the insertion sequence
d) Incorporating a tyrosine kinase gene into the insertion sequence
e) Incorporating an antibiotic resistance gene into the insertion sequence

Items 87-89

Match the type of hypersensitivity with its most common features.

a) Type I
b) Type II
c) Type III
d) Type IV
e) Types II and IV

87. Its synovial joints are primary targets of the reaction.

88. It is seen in hemolytic disease of the newborn.

89. It involves IgE.

90. Which of the following tracts contains axons of the pyramidal system which are destined for brainstem motor nuclei?

a) Nigrostriate tract
b) Mamillotegmental tract
c) Corticonuclear tract
d) Corticospinal tract
e) Central tegmental tract

USMLE step 1

BASIC MEDICAL SCIENCES

BOOK F TEST 2

TEST 2

Questions: 90 Time: 90 minutes

1. An 18 month-old black boy is brought to the emergency room with fever, cough and lethargy. The blood cultures obtained a day after the admission grew *Bordetella pertussis*. Which of the following statements regarding this bacteria is INCORRECT?

a) It is associated with a characteristic cough primarily in infants
b) It is produces a cytotoxin which damages ciliated tracheal cells
c) It is transmitted to humans by airborne droplets
d) It is invades underlying host tissue to reach the bloodstream
e) The blood smear of infected patient shows leukocytosis with predominantly lymphocytes

2. Recent research found that the cerebellar dentate nuclei were activated by motor tasks requiring sensory input but not by motor tasks not requiring sensory input. This experiment provides direct evidence that the cerebellum is involved in executing:

a) motor coordination
b) motor tasks for sensory discrimination
c) cognitive function
d) sensory perception
e) coordinated timing of motor tasks

3. A 60 year-old white female is seen in the office for loss of weight. The primary care physician ordered several tests including carcinoembriogenic antigen (CEA) and alpha-fetoprotein (AFP) in the blood. Which of the following statements regarding tumor immunity is CORRECT?

a) Malignant tumors never regress in human and animal models
b) In animal models, chemically-induced tumors often cross-react when induced by the same chemical
c) Virally-induced tumors seldom cross-react with one another when induced by the same chemical
d) Carcinoembryonic antigen is present in high levels in carcinomas of the colon, pancreas, breast, and liver, and is also present in normal adult serum
e) A high alpha-fetoprotein level indicates malignant hepatoma in 95% of cases

4. A 24-year-old woman develops severe diarrhea 36 hours after attending a picnic. A stool sample reveals neutrophils but no RBCs. Bacteria isolates include gram-negative rods which do not ferment lactose but produce H_2S. Which of the following is MOST likely the genus of this microorganism?

a) *Escherichia*
b) *Shigella*
c) *Salmonella*
d) *Campylobacter*
e) *Vibrio*

Items 5-7

Match the following neuroanatomy structures with its most appropriate functions and features.

a) Anterior pituitary
b) Posterior pituitary
c) Hypothalamus
d) Pineal gland
e) Basal ganglia

5. It is responsible for the synthesis of melatonin.

6. It has strong connections with the amygdala.

7. It may contain the corpora arenacea.

8. Each of the following are mechanisms to generate antibody diversity, EXCEPT:

a) combinatorial association of any V gene with any J gene with any D gene
b) point mutations in B cell chromosomes
c) enzymatic insertion of nucleotides at the junction between rearranged genes
d) imprecise joining of genes during DNA rearrangement
e) enzymatic alteration of the binding affinity of surface immunoglobulin

9. Two hours after eating a potluck meal featuring canned beans, omelets, and pork chops, several diners develop nausea, vomiting, and diarrhea. Which of the following organisms is the MOST likely cause of the outbreak?

a) *Staphylococcus aureus*
b) *Salmonella choleraesius*
c) *Clostridium perfringes*
d) *Clostridium difficile*
e) *Pseudomonas aeruginosa*

Items 10 - 13

The following is a diagram of a human spinal cord (see figure 3). Match the level of the lesion with its MOST likely clinical presentation.

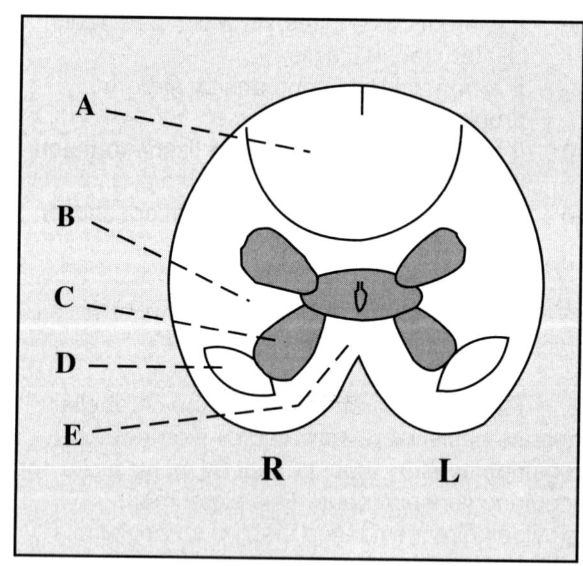

Figure 3 (Question 2.10)

10. A lesion here will result in a loss of pain and thermal sensation.

11. A lesion here will result in a loss of touch and pressure sensation.

12. A lesion here will result in spastic paralysis.

13. A lesion here will result in predominantly a contralateral deficit.

14. Each of the following is characteristic of an upper motor neuron syndrome EXCEPT:

a) increased muscle tone
b) hyperactive myotatic reflexes
c) affects limb muscles either contralateral or ipsilateral to the site of the lesion
d) extensor plantar reflex
e) pronounced muscular atrophy

15. A 14 month-old girl is brought to the clinic for dehydration secondary to severe diarrhea. The most likely viral agent responsible of this condition is:

a) Bunyavirus
b) Norwalk virus
c) Poliovirus
d) Vibrio parahaemolyticus
e) Rotavirus

16. Which of the following elements regulates muscle tautness to maintain sensitivity of muscle spindles?

a) Renshaw interneuron
b) Upper motor neuron
c) Golgi tendon organ
d) Alpha motoneuron
e) Gamma motoneuron

17. Each of the drugs below would directly prevent the synthesis of exotoxins in bacteria, EXCEPT:

a) chloramphenicol
b) erythromycin
c) tetracycline
d) streptomycin
e) trimethoprim

18. A 53 year old male with a history of alcoholism walks with an unstable gait, staggering stiff-leggedly. He is unable to slide the heel of one foot down the shin of the other leg without losing his balance. His upper limbs and speech are unaffected, and his blood-alcohol content is 0.03 mg/dL. What is the most likely site of degeneration in this patient's nervous system?

a) Gracile tract
b) Flocculonodular lobe
c) Anterior cerebellar lobe
d) Posterior cerebellar lobe
e) Cerebral cortex

19. Which of the following is the LEAST likely mechanism by which autoimmunity develops?

a) Diminished suppressor T cell function
b) Enhanced helper T cell function by a cross-reaction
c) Exit of antigenic self proteins from immunologically-privileged sites
d) Production of a blocking antibody to the estrogen receptor
e) Polyclonal B cell activation by Epstein-Barr virus

Items 20-22

Match the following types of hepatitis viruses with its MOST common features.

a) Hepatitis A virus (HAV)
b) Hepatitis B virus (HBV)
c) Hepatitis C virus (HCV)
d) Hepatitis D virus (HDV)
e) Hepatitis E virus (HEV)

20. A small RNA virus which cannot replicate independently.

21. About 10% of persons infected with this DNA virus become chronic carriers.

22. This enveloped RNA virus is the most common cause of posttransfusion hepatitis.

23. During a physical examination, a patient with a history of brain tumor is unable to recognize anything placed in the left superior quadrants (see diagram in figure 4). This defect is most likely due to a compression or mass effect at the:

a) optic chiasm
b) upper part of right geniculocalcarine tract
c) lower part of right geniculocalcarine tract
d) right lateral geniculate body
e) left striate area of the visual cortex

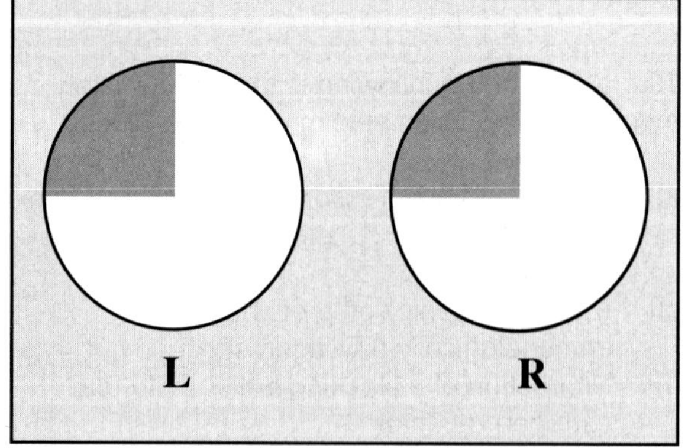

Figure 4 (Question 2.23)

Items 24-25

24. According the figure 5, what cell surface molecule is represented by the letter «A».

«APC» = antigen-presenting cell
bold arrowhead = antigen

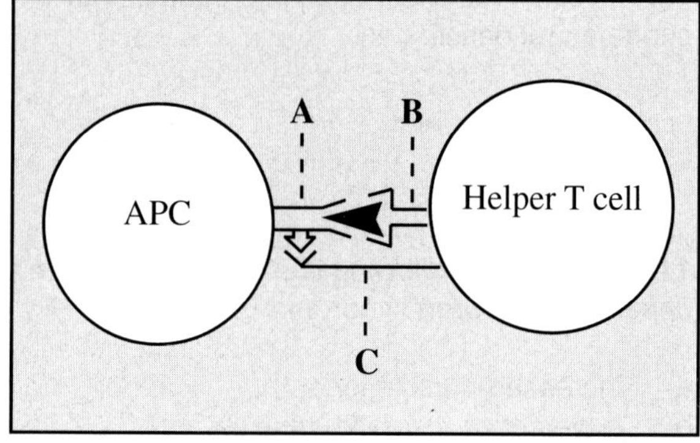

Figure 5 (Question 2.24)

a) CD3
b) CD4
c) CD8
d) MHC class I
e) MHC class II

25. The receptor depicted by letter «C» would be most likely to have affinity for which of the following human immunodeficiency (HIV) proteins:

a) gp41
b) gp120
c) p24
d) p31
e) p66

26. A 23 year-old white male is seen in the office with skin lesions seen in figure 6. You suspect a poxvirus infection. The following statements regarding this infection are correct, EXCEPT:

a) poxviruses have a linear double-stranded DNA genome
b) poxviruses are enveloped and are among the largest known viruses
c) poxviruses may promote neoplastic transformation after integration into host DNA
d) immunity to variola may be induced through inoculation with vaccinia virus
e) a poxvirus is responsible for molluscum contagioum

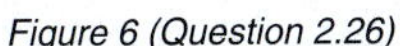

Figure 6 (Question 2.26)

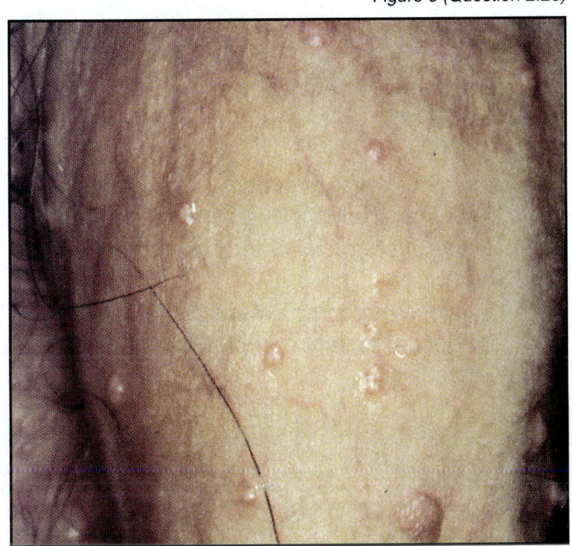

27. Each of the following statements regarding the functional histophysiology of the cerebellum is correct, EXCEPT:

a) the Purkinje cells excite the cerebellar nuclei
b) climbing fibers originate from the contralateral inferior olivary nucleus and contact Purkinje cells
c) the molecular layer of the cerebellar cortex contains most of the dendrites from the Purkinje cells
d) the cerebellar nuclei, from lateral to medial, are the dentate, interposite, and fastigial
e) in the cerebellar cortex, Golgi cells inhibit granule cells

28. During a physical exam, a 39 year-old man is injected intradermaly with a small amount of tuberculin antigen from *Mycobacterium tuberculosis*. Two days later, this area of skin becomes red and swollen. Which of the following statements contains the best interpretation of this phenomenon?

a) The man had never been exposed to *M. tuberculosis* prior to this test
b) The man has been exposed to *M. tuberculosis* in the past and may or may not have an active infection
c) The man has recently been exposed to *M. tuberculosis* and currently has an active infection
d) The man has recently been exposed to *M. tuberculosis* and is in the prodromal phase prior to the onset of infection
e) The redness and induration are due to immune complex formation

29. Which of the following is true of neoplastic transformation of virally infected cells?

a) Adenovirus protein R7 binds p53 and adenovirus protein p110 binds WT1
b) Poxvirus protein E3 binds RB1 and herpesvirus protein L1 binds abl
c) Adenovirus expresses an E1A protein which binds RB1 and a E1B protein which binds *N-ras*
d) Human papillomavirus (HPV) protein E6 binds p53 and E7 protein binds RB1
e) HPV protein E7 and adenovirus protein E1B both bind the *erbA* oncogene

30. A 56-year-old patient is seen in the office for severe headache, associated with meningeal signs and keratoconjunctivitis. Which of the following virus is most likely responsible for this clinical picture?

a) Human papilloma virus (HPV)
b) Epstein-Barr virus (EBV)
c) Cytomegalovirus (CMV)
d) Varicella-zoster virus (VZV)
e) Herpes simplex virus 1 (HSV1)

Items 31-32

Choose the most likely drug which has produced the effects in the patients below who are brought to the emergency room.

a) isoflurophate
b) morphine
c) scopolamine
d) d-tubocurarine
e) meperidine
f) phenylephrine

31. A 26 year-old female presents with motor weakness and difficulty breathing. She has difficulty moving her arms, legs, and head, and cannot move her fingers, toes, or extraocular muscles. Her speech is slurred and jaw movement is weak. Her pupils show mydriasis and respond to light sluggishly. Her blood pressure is 92/58 mmHg. She is conscious and has a clear sensorium.

32. A 31 year-old male who was agitated and delirious upon admission 20 minutes age is now drowsy and disoriented. His eyes show mydriasis and cycloplegia. His heart rate is 138 beats/minute, though he is not sweating. His mouth is very dry, and his temperature is slightly elevated at 38.2°C.

Items 33-34

A 6 month-old boy suffers from recurrent upper respiratory tract infections. He is congested and shows a mild facial hypoplasia. His serum immunoglobulins are within the normal range, but blood chemistry indicates hypocalcemia.

33. The disease most likely to present with these signs and symptoms is:

a) Severe Combined Immunodeficiency
b) Chediak-Higashi syndrome
c) Ataxia telangiectasia
d) DiGeorge syndrome
e) Wiskott-Aldrich syndrome

34. The immune deficiency seen in this patient is the result of:

a) congenital viral infection.
b) defective production of superoxide radicals.
c) failure of stem cell differentiation in bone marrow.
d) deficiency of complement components.
e) congenital absence of pharyngeal arch derivatives.

35. The pontine trigeminal nucleus transmits impulses from the face to the primary sensory cortex in which of the following manners?

a) Thermal sensation to the ipsilateral cortex
b) Pressure sensation to the ipsilateral cortex
c) Thermal sensation to the contralateral cortex
d) Pressure sensation to the contralateral cortex
e) Pressure and thermal sensation to the contralateral cortex

36. Which of the following statements concerning the envelope spikes* of paramyxoviruses is CORRECT?

*HA = hemagglutinin, NA = neuraminidas.

a) Only a fusion protein is present on the envelope spikes of mumps virus
b) All paramyxoviruses have HA and NA activity on their envelope spikes
c) Measles virus has an NA envelope spike but no HA envelope spike
d) Parainfluenza virus has HA and NA on the same envelope spike
e) Respiratory syncytial virus (RSV) and measles virus share the same envelope spikes

37. Each of the following cells or tissues develop from neural crest cells, EXCEPT:

a) adrenal cortex
b) dorsal root ganglia
c) parasympathetic ganglion cells
d) melanocytes
e) leptomeninges

38. Each of the following are facultative parasites, EXCEPT:

a) *Hymenolypus nana*
b) *Stronglyoides stercoralis*
c) *Naegleria*
d) *Hartmanella*
e) *Acanthamoeba*

Items 39-40

Match the appropriate protozoan parasite with the clinical descriptions below.

a) *Plasmodium falciparum*
b) *Plasmodium vivax*
c) *Trypanosoma cruzi*
d) *Trypanosoma gambiense*
e) *Leishmania donovani*

39. A South American white male presents with fever, periorbital swelling and syncope. The physical examination shows a mesocardial heart murmur. An EKG was obtained and shows a third degree atrial-ventricular heart block.

40. An African black male presents with headache and myalgia, as well as fever and chills which recur every 48 hours. Blood smear shows organisms in about 5% RBCs, at all stages of maturity; some organisms are banana-shaped.

41. Which of the following parasitic organisms is LEAST dependent upon environmental water to complete its life cycle?

a) *Diphylobothrium latum*
b) *Trichinella spiralis*
e) *Schistosoma mansoni*
d) *Paragonimus westermani*
e) *Anisakis*

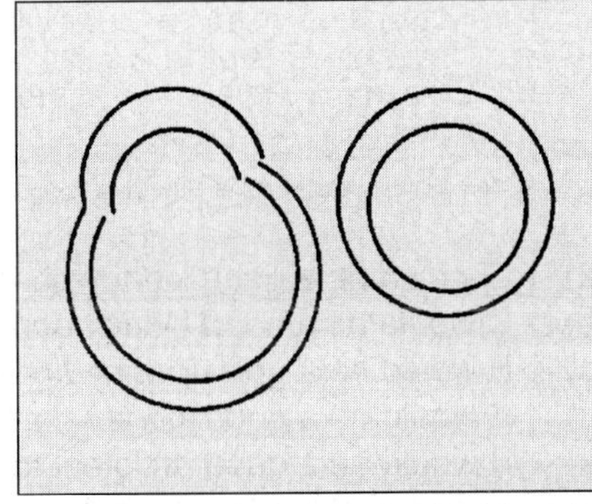

Figure 7 (Question 2.42)

Items 42-43

Match the MOST likely fungal infection in the following clinical presentations.

a) *Coccidioides*
b) *Cryptococcus*
c) *Histoplasma*
d) *Blastomyces*
e) *Aspergillus*

42. A 38 year-old woman living in Virginia develops a cough and ulcerated granulomas of the skin. A skin biopsy (see figure 7) shows doubly-refractive, broad-based yeast forms at 37°C, which later appear as a slender mold form when cultured at 20°C. She improves after a regimen of ketoconazole.

43. A 45 year-old pet-store employee on immunosuppressive drugs following an organ transplant develops symptoms of pneumonia, followed by headaches and changes in mental status. An India ink stain of spinal fluid shows yeast cells with a wide, unstained capsule.

44. Mixed lymphocyte reactions were done using cells from 4 different people. From the data in the table below, and assuming a good match for all other pertinent transplant antigens, which of the following would be expected?

Responders	A*	B*	C*	D*
A	332	24,976	512	547
B	39,871	455	26,689	14,003
C	28,370	19,099	389	219
D	32,042	16,114	3,819	502

*Irradiated stimulator cells (3H thymidine incorporation in DPM)

a) C would be a good kidney donor for D
b) D would be a good kidney donor for C
c) B would be a good kidney donor for A
d) A would be a good kidney donor for B
e) B would be a good recipient for a kidney from any of the potential donors above

Items 45-47

The following diagram (see figure 8) represents the somatosensory pathway by which pressure sensation travels from the ankle to the cerebral cortex. (Use the following options for items 45 and 46).

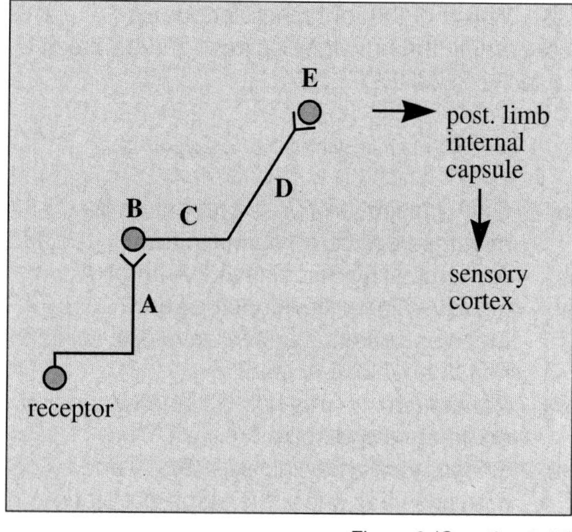

Figure 8 (Question 2.45)

a) Cuneate tract
b) Gracile tract
c) Medial lemniscus
d) Spinothalamic tract
e) Dorsolateral tract of Lissauer

45. What is the name of the tract at «A»?

46. If the fibers decussate at «C», what tract is represented by «D»?

47. Which part of the thalamus is represented by «E» in figure 8?

a) Ventral anterior
b) Ventral lateral
c) Ventral posterior medial
d) Ventral posterior lateral
e) Medial dorsal

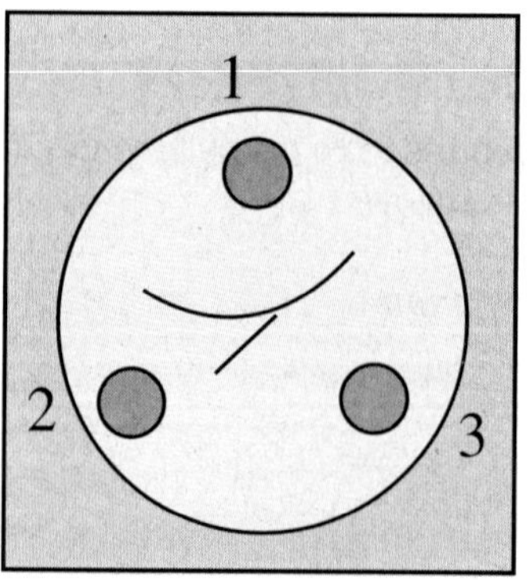

Figure 9 (Question 2.48)

48. Figure 9 shows an Ouchterlony double gel-diffusion assay. Well 1 contains goat antibody against human serum albumin. Which of the following antigens are most likely present in wells 2 and 3?

	Well 2	Well 3
a)	Human IgG	Bovine IgG
b)	Human albumin	Bovine serum
c)	Bovine albumin	Human IgG
d)	Human serum	Bovine IgG
e)	Bovine albumin	Human albumin

Items 49-51

Match the following immunodeficiency diseases with their most common clinical features.

a) Chronic granulomatous disease
b) Hereditary angioedema
c) Common variable hypogammaglobulinemia
d) Wiskott-Aldrich syndrome
e) Bruton's agammaglobulinemia

49. A 38 year-old white male who presents recurrent bacterial infections beginning as a teenager.

50. A 12 month-old white male with normal IgG levels, who fails to mount IgM responses to bacterial capsules.

51. A 35 year-old white female who lacks C1 esterase inhibitor.

Items 52-53

Gram-stain and the bacteria wall.

Item 52

Which of the following lists the proper sequence of reagents used in a gram stain?

a) Safranin, then acetone, then crystal violet, then iodine
b) Crystal violet, then acetone, then iodine, then safranin
c) Safranin, then iodine, then crystal violet, then acetone
d) Safranin, then iodine, then acetone, then crystal violet
e) Crystal violet, then iodine, then acetone, then safranin

Item 53

Which of the following statements regarding the bacteria cell wall is CORRECT?

a) Teichoic acids are present in gram-negative but not gram-positive cell walls
b) Gram-positive cell walls have relatively more lipopolysaccharide (LPS) than gram-negative cell walls
c) Gram-positive cell walls have relatively more lipoprotein and phospholipid than do gram-negative cell walls
d) Capsules are present on gram-negative but not gram-positive cell walls
e) Gram-positive cell walls have a thicker layer of peptidoglycan than gram-negative cell walls

54. Each of the following correctly pairs bacterial organisms with their appearance following a gram stain, EXCEPT:

	Genus	Morphology	Color
a)	*Vibrio*	curved rod	red
b)	*Neisseria*	cocci in clusters	red
c)	*Staphylococcus*	cocci in clusters	blue
d)	*Bacillis*	square-ended rod	blue
e)	*Corynebacterium*	club-shaped rod	blue

55. The neurotransmitter which is found in the greatest percentage of the brain synapses is:

a) GABA
b) Acetylcholine
c) Norepinephrine
d) Dopamine
e) Glutamate

56. Which of the following types of RNA virus is LEAST likely to encode a polymerase enzyme in its genome?

a) Single-stranded, nonsegmented, positive polarity
b) Single-stranded, nonsegmented, negative polarity
c) Single-stranded, segmented, negative polarity
d) Single-stranded, diploid, positive polarity
e) Double-stranded, segmented

57. Dementia:

a) is only vascular in origin
b) risk factors for Alzheimer's type include female gender, history of head injury, and Down's syndrome
c) after the age of seventy, the risk for developing this condition declines
d) is reversible in 50 % of the patients if treatment is initiated in a timely fashion
e) involves memory impairment with shifting levels of consciousness

58. Each of the following are endogenous fibrinolytic substances present in humans, EXCEPT:

a) plasmin
b) urokinase
c) streptokinase
d) heparin
e) antithrombin III

59. Several organs receive both sympathetic and parasympathetic innervation. At which of the following sites does parasympathetic tone predominate?

a) Sinoatrial (SA) node
b) Cardiac ventricle
c) Arterioles
d) Veins
e) Sweat glands

60. Each of the following statements apply to human fluids (such as blood) flowing through a tube (such as a blood vessel), EXCEPT:

a) the apparent viscosity of the fluid increases as the diameter of the vessel increases.
b) an increase in the pressure gradient between the ends of the tube will lead to an increase in the flow.
c) the flow through the tube increases as the radius of the tube increases.
d) as the apparent viscosity of the fluid increases, the flow through the tube decreases.
e) the flow through the tube increases as the length of the tube increases.

61. Aside from motor vehicle accidents, which type of accident typically accounts for the greatest number of fatalities in a given year?

a) Poisoning
b) Firearms
c) Fires or burns
d) Falls
e) Drowning

62. In the clinic, you suspect that your patient has an acute occlusion of the common carotid arteries. The most common finding of this condition is:

a) a decrease in heart rate
b) a decrease in blood pressure
c) a decrease in vagus nerve discharge
d) a decrease in sympathetic nerve discharge
e) an increase in blood flow through the facial artery

63. The following statements regarding the accidental deaths in the U.S. are correct, EXCEPT:

a) about half of fatally injured drivers are legally intoxicated
b) between the ages of 1 and 37, accidents are the leading cause of death
c) accidental death are most frequent on Mondays during the winter
d) per capita income is negatively correlated with motor vehicle deaths, but unrelated to deaths from falls
e) the overall rural accident death rate is higher than the urban rate

64. The condition that tends to favor the outflow of fluid from capillaries is:

a) an increase in the reflection coefficient
b) a decrease in capillary hydrostatic pressure
c) an increase in capillary osmotic pressure
d) an increase in interstitial osmotic pressure
e) an increase in interstitial hydrostatic pressure

65. A true statement regarding the suicide tendency in the U.S. is:

a) most (over 90%) people who commit suicide have a diagnosable mental disorder
b) females attempt and complete suicide more frequently than males
c) suicide is the leading cause of death among teenagers
d) people rarely (under 10%) see a physician before attempting suicide
e) after age 25, the suicide rate decreases with increasing age

66. Which of the following personality disorder patients are most likely to attempt and/or complete suicide?

	Attempt	**Complete**
a)	Paranoid	Schizotypal
b)	Narcissistic	Passive-aggressive
c)	Obsessive-compulsive	Borderline
d)	Histrionic	Schizoid
e)	Borderline	Antisocial

Items 67 - 69

A 2-year-old girl has experienced severe diarrhea for three days. Her blood gases and electrolytes are measured as follows (reference ranges in parentheses):

Sodium	130 mEq/L	(133-145)
Potassium	3.0 mEq/L	(3.5-5)
Chloride	120 mEq/L	(100-112)
Bicarbonate	5 mEq/L	(normal = 24)
PaCO2	16	(normal = 40)
[H+]	77 nEq/L	(normal = 40)
pH	7.23	(7.35-7.45)

67. What is the patient's acid-base disturbance?

a) Metabolic acidosis
b) Metabolic alkalosis
c) Respiratory acidosis
d) Respiratory alkalosis
e) Mixed acid-base disturbance

68. What is the patient's anion gap?

a) 2
b) 5
c) 8
d) 10
e) 12

69. Which of the following would be the most appropriate to include in the initial treatment of this patient?

a) Encourage hyperventilation
b) Administer 100% oxygen
c) Administer an anticholingeric agent
d) Intravenous bicarbonate
e) Intravenous sodium lactate

70. Health insurances:

a) over one third of Americans have no health insurance
b) Medicare is a program for low income groups and is funded primarily by state governments
c) Medicaid is a program for persons over age 65 and is federally funded
d) Medicaid is a program for low income groups and is partially funded by state governments
e) health maintenance organizations (HMOs) are available only to employed persons and are partially funded by the federal government

Items 71-73

A 25 year-old white female was seen in the hospital for a work up of posterior cervical lymphadenopathy. She presented with several enlarged lymph nodes, firm, non-tender and fixed to deep layers in both sides of the neck. A surgical biopsy of the lymph nodes was obtained (see figure 10a).

71. The arrow in the figure indicates:

a) a normal macrophage
b) a Reed-Sternberg cell
c) a multinucleated normal inflammatory cell
d) a cyst
e) a parasite

72. The most likely diagnosis is:

a) Leishmaniasis
b) Acute leukemia
c) Hodgkin's lymphoma
d) Chronic leukemia
e) hyperplastic lymph nodes

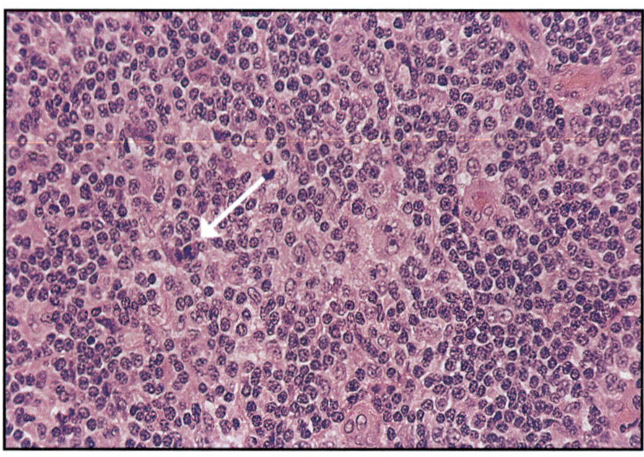

Figure 10a (Question 2.71)

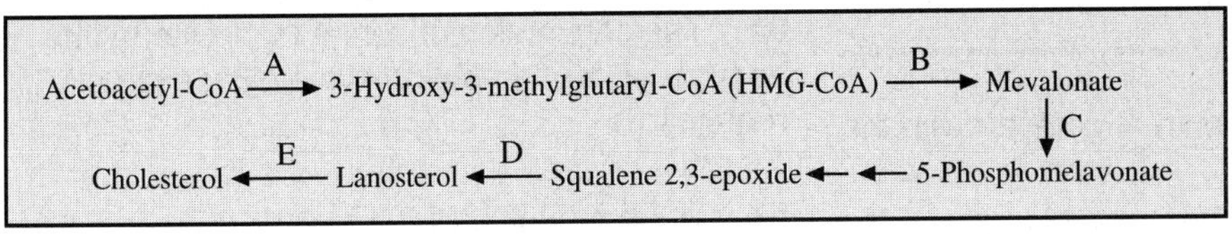

Acetoacetyl-CoA —A→ 3-Hydroxy-3-methylglutaryl-CoA (HMG-CoA) —B→ Mevalonate

Mevalonate —C→ 5-Phosphomelavonate

5-Phosphomelavonate → → Squalene 2,3-epoxide —D→ Lanosterol —E→ Cholesterol

Figure 10b (Question 2.78)

73. Which of the following statements regarding this disease is INCORRECT?

a) The spleen is involved in one-third of the cases at the time of diagnosis
b) The lymph nodes are usually firm or rubbery with «fish flesh» appearance
c) The bone marrow can be infiltrated with an osteolytic appearance
d) At autopsy most patients present with liver infiltration
e) A multifocal infiltration of malignant plasma cells in the bone marrow is often seen

74. The use of lithium is commonly associated with side effects. Four of the following adverse responses are experienced by about one-third of the patients with lithium levels within the therapeutic serum range. Which side effect is relatively rare among these patients?

a) Polyuria
b) Gastrointestinal disturbance
c) Edema
d) Muscle weakness
e) Leukocytosis

75. Which of the following bones does NOT develop entirely from a cartilagenous model?

a) Parietal bone
b) Ethmoid bone
c) Ephenoid bone
d) Temporal bone
e) Occipital bone

Items 76-77

On a routine physical exam, a 62 year-old woman is found to have a serum calcium of 7.4 mg/dL (normal = 9 - 10.5). Radiographic imaging shows attenuated, thin lamellar bone. A metabolic disease of bone is suspected.

76. The patient most likely has:

a) osteopetrosis
b) osteoporosis
c) osteomalacia
d) ankylosing spondylitis
e) osteomyelitis

77. Which of the metabolic derangements below is LEAST likely to be contributing to this patient's condition?

a) Subnormal levels of parathyroid hormone
b) Subnormal levels of 1,25 OH2 vitamin D3
c) Subnormal levels of estrogen
d) Subnormal levels of calcitonin
e) Inadequate exposure to sunlight

78. In the abbreviated pathway shown in figure 10b, which enzyme catalyzes the first committed step of cholesterol biosynthesis?

79. Each of the following vitamins has shared structural features with the monoterpene compound shown in the figure 10c, EXCEPT:

a) vitamin A
b) vitamin K
c) vitamin C
d) vitamin D
e) vitamin E

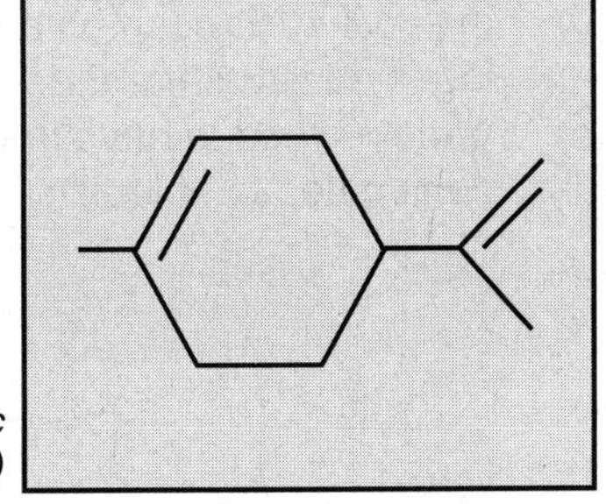

Figure 10c (Question 2.79)

Items 80-82

Match the appropriate vitamin or cofactor with the statements below.

a) Niacin
b) Thiamine (vitamin B1)
c) Riboflavin (vitamin B2)
d) Pyridoxine (vitamin B6)
e) Cyanocobalamin (vitamin B12)

80. Cofactor for dehydrogenase enzymes; deficiency results in dermatitis, dementia, and diarrhea (pellagra).

81. Required for the methylation of homocysteine to methionine and the conversion of methylmalonyl CoA to succinyl CoA; synthesized by intestinal flora; deficiency results in megaloblastic anemia and peripheral neuropathy.

82. Needed for transamination and decarboxylation reactions; deficiency state may arise from alcoholism or drug therapy (oral contraceptives, isoniazide).

83. Each of the following statements is TRUE regarding protein metabolism, EXCEPT:

a) marasmus is a combination of protein and caloric deficiency, while kwashiorkor results from a deficiency of protein in a diet relatively high in carbohydrates.
b) arginine, lysine, and valine are all required in the diets of mammals.
c) alanine, cysteine, and asparagine are all considered nonessential amino acids.
d) in positive nitrogen balance, the nitrogen ingested is greater than that excreted
e) proteins tend to have longer half-lifes when conjugated to ubiquitin.

84. The conversion of serine to glycine by the enzyme serine transhydroxymethylase directly requires:

a) alpha-ketoglutarate and S-adenosylmethionine (SAM).
b) deoxythymidylate monophosphate (dTMP) and NADPH.
c) pyridoxal phosphate and tetrahydrofolate
d) ascorbic acid and ATP.
e) avidin and phosphoribosylpyrophosphate

85. Each of the following correctly pairs a signaling molecule with its amino acid precursor EXCEPT:

	Precursor	Product
a)	arginine	nitric oxide
b)	tyrosine	thyroxine (T_4)
c)	tyrosine	dopamine
d)	histidine	serotonin
e)	glutamate	GABA*

* Gamma-aminobutyric acid

86. 5-Phosphoribosylamine (PRA) is an intermediate in the biosynthesis of:

a) hemoglobin
b) aliphatic amino acids
c) purines
d) pyrimidines
e) cholesterol

87. Which of the following statements is true concerning the regulation of the lactose (*lac*) operon in prokaryotes?

a) The repressor binds the promotor, and the inducer binds the operator
b) The repressor binds the operator, and the inducer binds the promotor
c) The repressor binds the promotor, and the inducer binds the repressor
d) The repressor binds the operator, and the inducer binds the repressor
e) The repressor and the inducer both compete for binding sites on the promotor

88. The adrenergic receptor has seven hydrophobic regions which function as transmembrane domains (TMDs). The receptor is anchored in the membrane in a translocation process which is coincident with translation, and the initial signal peptide is cleaved. Given this information, the topology of such a receptor will be such that:

a) the N-terminus is more likely than the C-terminus to aid in binding external ligands
b) the N-terminus is more likely than the C-terminus to aid in intracellular signal transduction
c) the N- and C-termini are both located on the external cell surface
d) the N- and C-termini are both located in the cytosol
e) the N- and C-termini consist of start- and stop-transfer peptide signals, respectively, and thus are located within the membrane

89. The enzyme ribonucleotide diphosphate reductase (rNDP) is required for the ultimate conversion of:

a) adenine to guanine
b) thymidine to uracil
c) nucleotide diphosphates to nucleotide monophosphates
d) ADP to nicotinamide-adenine dinucleotide (NAD+)
e) RNA bases to DNA bases

90. Each of the following processes occurs at least partially in the mitochondrion, EXCEPT:

a) biosynthesis of ketone bodies
b) fatty acid biosynthesis
c) fatty acid degradation
d) generation of urea from ammonia
e) the citric acid cycle

USMLE step 1

BASIC MEDICAL SCIENCES

BOOK F TEST 3

Questions: 90 Time: 90 minutes

1. Interleukin-1 is produced primarily by which of the following cells?

a) Lymphocytes
b) Macrophages
c) Mast cells
d) Natural killer cells
e) Polymorphonuclear neutrophils (PMNs)

2. The MOST impaired mechanism of immunity in a patient with severe combined immunodeficiency (SCID) is:

a) natural killer cell function
b) toxin neutralization
c) production of acute phase proteins
d) neutrophil phagocytosis
e) complement-mediated lysis

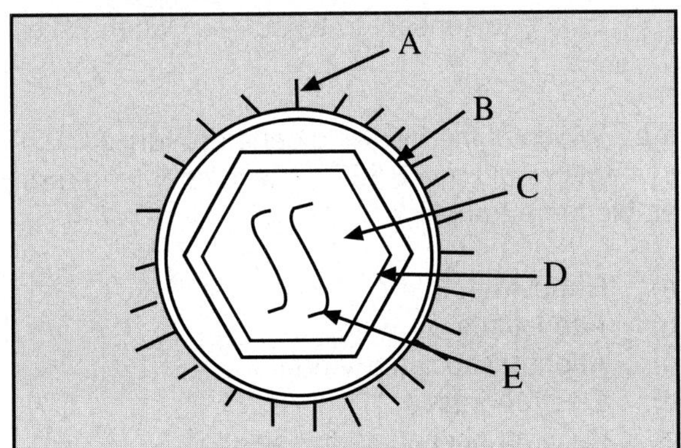

Figure 11 (Question 3.3)

Items 3-5

Refer to the diagram showing an icosahedral virus in cross-section (see figure 11).

3. It contains elements manufactured using a host chromosome sequence.

4. It is first to be reproduced following the eclipse phase.

5. It is most likely to mediate adsorption.

6. The symptom of angina pectoris is relieved by nitroglycerin because:

a) it has a negative inotropic effect
b) it has a positive chronotropic effect
c) it possesses analgesic properties
d) it dissolves atherosclerotic plaques
e) it decreases ventricular wall tension

7. Which of the following drugs is NOT used to treat tuberculosis?

a) Isoniazid
b) Dapsone
c) Rifampin
d) Ethambutol
e) Pyrazinamide

8. The «sick role» as described by Parsons includes two rights and two obligations for patients. The two rights are:

a) accepting responsibility and choosing a physician
b) choosing a physician and relaxed role obligations
c) blamelessness and relaxed role obligations
d) receiving care regardless of ability to pay and blamelessness
e) choosing a physician and receiving care regardless of ability to pay.

Items 9-10

Select the best answer from the list below.

a) DNA footprinting
b) Mobility shift DNA binding assay
c) Oligo-nucleotide mutagenesis
d) Linker scanning mutagenesis
e) Enzyme-linked immunosorbant assay (ELISA)

9. Alters a DNA sequence in a defined way.

10. It can be used to locate the specific binding site of a protein on DNA.

11. Under physiological conditions, which of the following is most likely to increase the rate of diffusion through a cell membrane?

a) Decreasing the temperature
b) Decreasing the viscosity of the membrane
c) Increasing the size of the diffusible molecule
d) Decreasing the concentration gradient across the membrane
e) Increasing the phospholipid content of the membrane

12. Which of the following is CORRECT regarding the antibiotic sulbactam?

a) It is an extended spectrum ß-lactam drug.
b) It is a third generation cephalosporin.
c) It is best used in combination with chloramphenicol.
d) It is a ß-lactamase inhibitor.
e) It is a sulfonamide.

13. Which of the following statements regarding the circumstances surrounding death is CORRECT?

a) Cortical death occurs when the brainstem ceases to function
b) In the U.S., consent for organ donations is presumed
c) The autopsy rate is increasing in U.S. hospitals
d) In about 16% of autopsies of older adults, no specific disease process is found which would cause death in a younger person
e) Most families become offended and will refuse to consent to an autopsy when asked

14. Which of the following gene delivery systems would be LEAST likely to offer long-term stable gene transfer?

a) Retrovirus
b) Adenovirus
c) Adeno-associated Virus
d) Electroporation
e) Calcium-phosphate transfection

15. The hormone responsible for the libido in females is MOST likely:

a) ovarian estrogen
b) ovarian androgen
c) adrenal estrogen
d) adrenal androgen
e) luteinizing hormone

Figure 12 (Question 3.16)

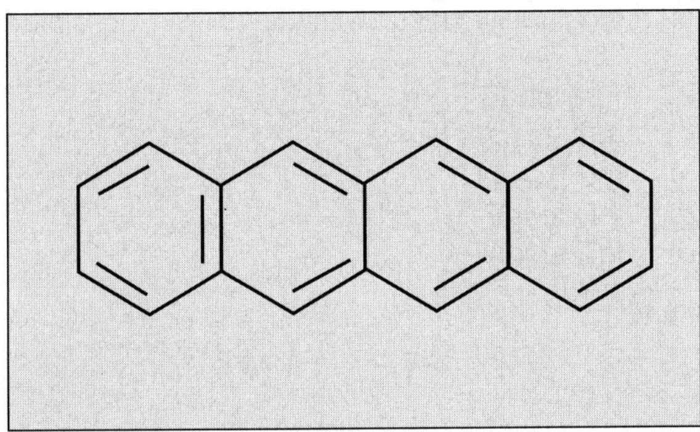

16. The chemical structure shown in figure 12 would be most likely found in a drug belonging to which of the following classes?

a) Antihelminthic
b) Antimicrobial
c) Antineoplastic
d) Antipsychotic
e) Anti-inflammatory

17. A 39 year-old man seeks medical attention because of intermittent episodes of uncontrollable, violent jerking movements of his right shoulders, upper arms, and thighs. The CNS structure MOST likely damaged in this patient is:

a) globus pallidus
b) substantia nigra
c) caudate nucleus
d) putamen
e) subthalamic nucleus

18. Each of the following autoimmune diseases are correctly matched with the antigen to which autoantibodies are produced, EXCEPT:

	Disease	Antigen
a)	Myasthenia gravis	ß-adrenergic receptor
b)	rheumatoid arthritis	immunoglobulin G
c)	systemic lupus erythematosus	double-stranded DNA
d)	rheumatic fever	cardiac myosin
e)	Hashimoto's thyroiditis	thyroglobulin

19. A 39 year-old white male is admitted to the hospital for chest pain and tachyrhythmia. A viral infection with pericarditis was documented. Which of the viruses below is MOST often the cause of this patient's condition?

a) Coronavirus
b) Rotavirus
c) Coxsackievirus
d) Influenzavirus
e) Togavirus

20. The posterolateral part of the frontal lobe (orbital gyri) is most likely involved in:

a) optokinetic nystagmus
b) judgment and calculation
c) audition
d) olfaction
e) taste

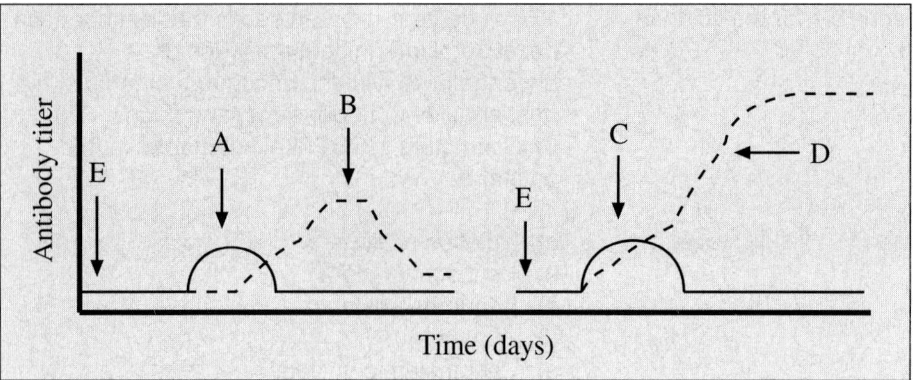

Figure 13 (Question 3.21)

Items 21-22

Refer to the graph below regarding the kinetics of the immune response (see figure 13).

21. Which curve indicates the IgG response upon the first exposure to an antigen?

22. Which curve indicates the IgM response upon a second exposure to the same antigen?

23. Which virus is surrounded by an envelope?

a) Parvovirus
b) Flavivirus
c) Calicivirus
d) Reovirus
e) Adenovirus

24. In an experimental model for ocular dominance plasticity, covering an eye early in the life of a mammal is most likely to have which of the following effects?

a) Degeneration of the optic tract of the covered eye
b) Bitemporal hemianopsia
c) A visual cortex which responds only to the eye which was not covered
d) A visual cortex which responds in exaggerated fashion to the eye which was covered
e) Processing of visual information from both eyes solely in the contralateral visual cortex

25. Due to the order of heavy chain genes, which of the following examples of immunoglobulin class switching is NOT possible?

a) IgM to IgD
b) IgG_3 to IgG_2
c) IgG_4 to IgA_2
d) IgD to IgE
e) IgE to IgA_1

26. A transcriptional factor has been identified which arrests the maturation of a cell which manufactures myelin in the peripheral nervous system. Which of the following would most likely result from a DECREASE in the intracellular levels of this factor?

a) A developmental delay of oligodendrocytes at the promyelin stage
b) A developmental delay of Schwann cells at the promyelin stage
c) Progression from the promyelin stage to the myelin stage in oligodendrocytes
d) Progression from the promyelin stage to the myelin stage in Schwann cells
e) An increase in myelination by microglia

Items 27-29

Refer to the following diagram (see figure 14) of a skeletal muscle sarcomere.

27. It is made of alpha actinin.

28. This band disappears during muscle contraction.

29. It is made of myosin.

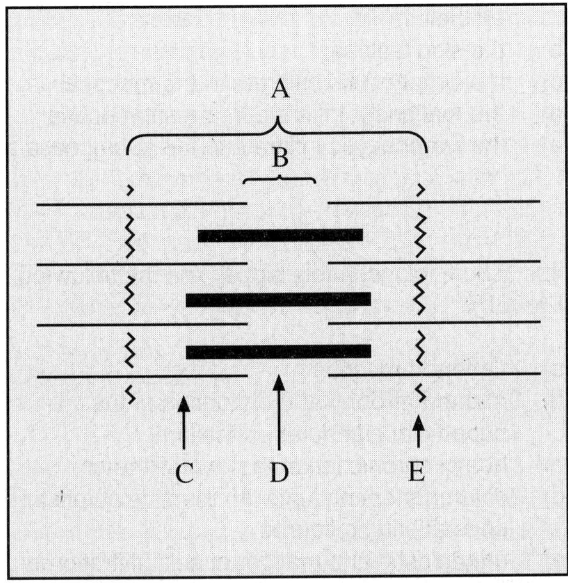

Figure 14 (Question 3.27)

30. A woman strikes her elbow on a desk top and feels a tingling sensation in her hand; she comments that she has hit her «funny bone.» The structure most likely to be responsible for this sensation is the:

a) Radial nerve
b) Ulnar nerve
c) Olecranon process
d) Medial epicondyle
e) Tendinous origin of the flexor digitorum superficialis

Items 31-32

a) Clomiphene
b) Mestranol
c) Tamoxifen
d) Ethinyl estradiol
e) Norethindrone

31. Useful in treating some forms of breast cancer.

32. A 29 year-old woman delivers triplets after having been on a regimen of this drug.

33. The antidepressant drug fluoxetine selectively inhibits the reuptake of which of the following neurotransmitters?

a) Dopamine
b) Norepinepherine
c) Serotonin
d) GABA
e) Acetylcholine

34. Which of the following divisions of the nervous system are responsible for the penile erection and ejaculation in the male?

	Erection	Ejaculation
a)	sympathetic	somatic
b)	parasympathetic	somatic
c)	somatic	sympathetic
d)	parasympathetic	sympathetic
e)	sympathetic	parasympathetic

35. Fibers of which of the following muscles are MOST likely to be cut by a superficial incision in the upper back?

a) Iliocostalis
b) Multifidus
c) Longissimus
d) Splenius
e) Semispinalis

36. Which of the following trends would be expected in a patient one month after beginning treatment with captopril?

	plasma aldosterone	plasma renin	plasma angiotensin II
a)	increased	increased	increased
b)	decreased	decreased	decreased
c)	increased	decreased	decreased
d)	decreased	increased	decreased
e)	decreased	decreased	increased

Items 37-40

A 62 year-old white female is seen for chronic watery diarrhea for the last 4 years. A biopsy of the transverse colon is obtained (see figure 15).

37. The histopathological findings are compatible with:

a) lymphoma
b) Crohn's disease
c) collagenous colitis
d) Adenocarcinoma
e) none of the above

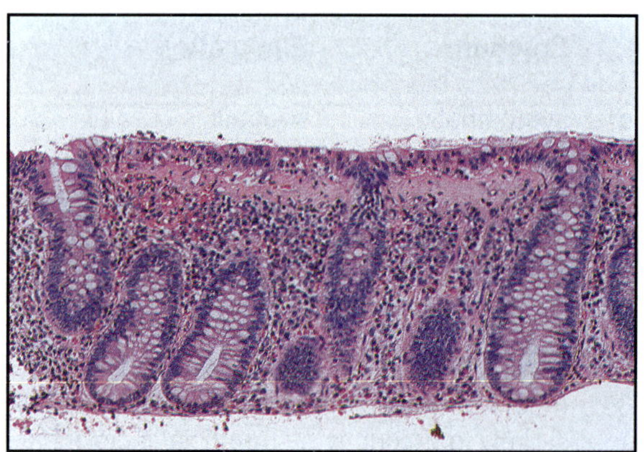

Figure 15 (Question 3.37)

38. The etiology of this condition is MOST likely:

a) mechanic lesion of the mucosa
b) autoimmune
c) neoplastic
d) infectious
e) genetic

39. The histopathological finding typical of this disease is:

a) the collagenous band beneath the surface epithelium
b) the skip lesions
c) the lymphocytic infiltrate in the mucosa
d) the malignant infiltrate in the submucosa
e) the lymphocytic infiltrate in the submucosa

40. The findings in this biopsy are the following, EXCEPT:

a) flattened mucosa
b) marked atrophy and distorsion of the superficial glandular epithelium
c) heavy chronic inflammatory infiltration
d) columnar epithelium with reactive atypia and several mitotic figures
e) metaplastic and malignant cell infiltration of the submucosa

Items 41-42

An antibody-based test for HIV infection is reported to have a sensitivity of 90% and a specificity of 80%. Ten thousand people from a population with a 10% incidence of HIV volunteer to be tested.

41. How many of these people will have a false positive test?

a) 100
b) 800
c) 900
d) 1700
e) 1800

42. Which of the following parameters is the HIGHEST in percentage for this population and this test?

a) Positive predictive value
b) Negative predictive value
c) Sensitivity
d) Specificity
e) Incidence of HIV

43. In a psychiatric hospital, arm restraints are removed when a patient behaves in a calm manner. This is an example of:

a) Habituation
b) Sensitization
c) Positive reinforcement
d) Negative reinforcement
e) Punishment

44. Intravenous sodium lactate can reproduce the symptoms of which of the following disorders?

a) Major depression
b) Bipolar disorder, manic episode
c) Panic disorder
d) Schizophreniform disorder
e) Post-traumatic stress disorder

Items 45-46

Figure 16 shows a section of fetal calvaria stained with an antibody against collagenase.

45. The blue-staining cells, which are responsible for the production of the surrounding matrix, are most likely:

a) osteoblasts
b) osteoclasts
c) osteocytes
d) chondrocytes
e) fibroblasts

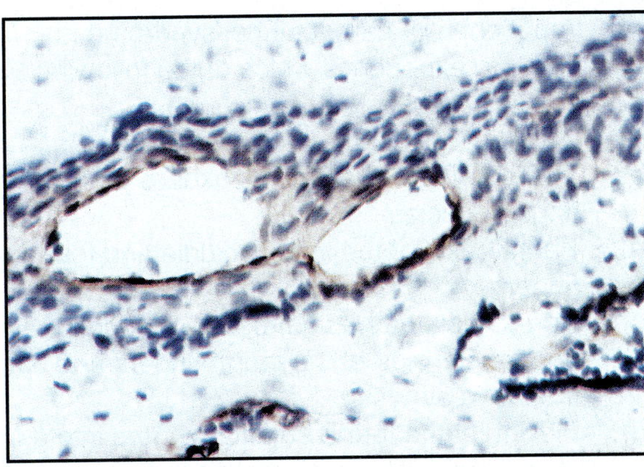

Figure 16 (Question 3.45)

46. Each of the following statements regarding normal bone is correct, EXCEPT:

a) osteoclasts are derived from hematopoietic precursors and mediate bone resorption.
b) osteoblasts mediate both bone formation and bone resorption.
c) osteocytes are surrounded by matrix but are able to receive nutrients through a canalicular system.
d) in the adult skeleton, there is relatively more trabecular bone than compact bone.
e) the inorganic matrix of bone is comprised primarily of calcium and phosphate.

Items 47-48

A third year medical student is instructed to perform a physical examination on a patient with a history of «carpal tunnel syndrome.»

47. This syndrome is produced by involvement of the:

a) median nerve and flexor retinaculum
b) median nerve and extensor retinaculum
c) radial nerve and flexor retinaculum
d) radial nerve and extensor retinaculum
e) ulnar nerve and extensor retinaculum

48. A patient with carpal tunnel syndrome is most likely to experience which of the following symptoms?

a) Flexion of the wrist and weakness of the finger muscles
b) Paresthesia of the index, middle and fourth fingers
c) Paresthesia of the thumb, index, middle, and medial side of the fourth fingers and thenar weakness
d) Flexion of the fourth and fifth fingers into a claw-like posture and weakness and paresthesia over the hypothenar region
e) Intermittent pain and paralysis of the hand

49. A hypertensive 52-year-old white male was started on drug A. The following laboratory values were obtained prior to and one week after the initiation of treatment with drug A (normal values in parentheses):

	Prior to A	**1 wk after A**
Serum Sodium (136-145 mEq/l)	140	137
Serum Potassium (3.5-5 mEq/l)	4.5	3.2
Serum Uric Acid (2.5-8 mg%)	6.0	8.8
Fasting blood glucose (75-115 mg%)	97	125
Arterial blood pH (7.35-7.45)	7.40	7.48

Drug A is MOST likely:

a) furosemide
b) captopril
c) minoxidil
d) hydrochlorothiazide
e) reserpine

50. Each of the following are functions of microsomal cytochrome P450, EXCEPT:

a) oxidation of phenobarbitol
b) oxidation of amphetamine
c) deamination of epinephrine
d) hydroxylation of cholesterol
e) adrenal steroidogenesis

51. The defense mechanisms that are MOST closely associated with obsessive-compulsive disorder are:

a) isolation and undoing
b) regression and splitting
c) splitting and undoing
d) displacement and conversion
e) displacement and introjection

52. What are the primary sources of testosterone and spermatocytes in the male?

	Testosterone	**Spermatocytes**
a)	Leydig cell	seminal vesicles
b)	Sertoli cell	Leydig cell
c)	Sertoli cell	seminal vesicle
d)	Leydig cell	Sertoli cell
e)	prostate gland	tunica albuginea

53. Which of the following statements regarding the chordae tendinae is CORRECT?

a) They are involved in the rapid conduction of electrical impulses from the atrioventricular (AV) node.
b) They help to prevent the cusps of the tricuspid valve from collapsing back into the right atrium.
c) They help prevent ballooning of the aortic valve into the left ventricle.
d) They anchor the pulmonic valve to the interventricular septum.
e) They are attached to atrial papillary muscles.

54. Each of the following situations are indications for an ethics consultation, EXCEPT:

a) foregoing lifesustaining treatment
b) writing a do-not-resuscitate (DNR) order
c) evaluating the validity of an advance directive
d) assessing patient decision-making capacity
e) deciding who should perform an autopsy

55. Which of the following hormones is MOST responsible for stimulating the production of androgen-binding protein (ABP)?

a) Follicle-Stimulating Hormone (FSH)
b) Luteinizing Hormone (LH)
c) Testosterone
d) Androstenedione
e) Cortisol

56. The artery that does NOT originate from the celiac trunk is:

a) left gastric
b) splenic
c) hepatic
d) gastroduodenal
e) superior mesenteric

Items 57-59

A 6 year-old white boy is seen in a medical office for failure to thrive, after his mother started cereals and other food products in his daily meals. A biopsy of the small intestine was performed (see figure 17).

57. This disease may:

a) present with malnutrition
b) present complications like lymphoma
c) present with ulcerative jejunitis
d) develop other solid gastrointestinal tumors
e) all the above are correct

58. The intervention that MOST likely can improve his condition is:

a) antibiotics
b) steroids
c) salt-free diet
d) gluten-free diet
e) radiation of his abdomen

59. The hallmark histopathological findings of this condition are the following, EXCEPT:

a) blunting of villi
b) disappearance of villi
c) damaged epithelial cells on the mucosal surface
d) neoplasic infiltration of mucosa and deeper layers
e) increased cellularity of the lamina propria but not of the deeper layers

Figure 17 (Question 3.57)

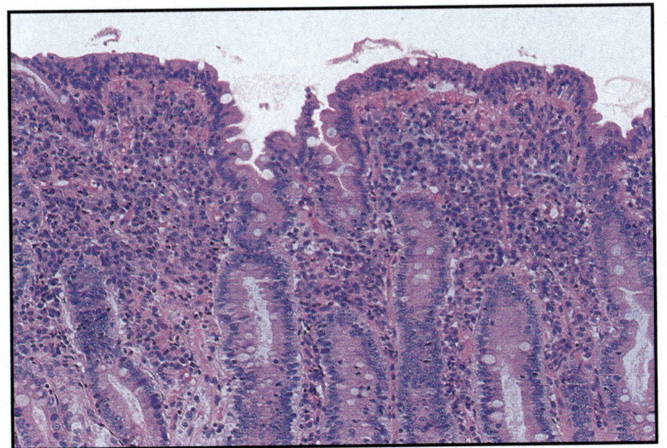

Figure 18 (Question 3.60)

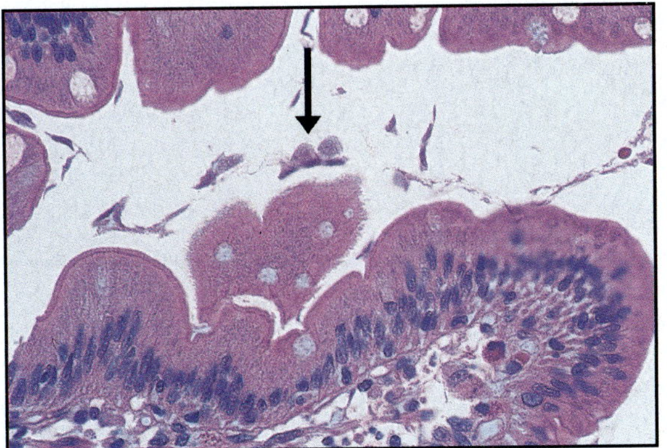

Items 60-62

A 36 year-old white male after returning from a camping trip, presents with abdominal bloating with nausea, anorexia, and watery diarrhea. An endoscopy was performed and biopsies were taken from the small intestine (see figure 18).

60. The most likely cause of this condition is:

a) inflammatory bowel disease
b) lymphoma
c) Giardiasis
d) food poisoning
e) none of the above

61. The arrow in the picture represents:

a) *Mycobacteria TB*
b) trophozoites
c) macrophages
d) reactive lymphocytes T
e) reactive lymphocytes B

62. The most likely mechanism of diarrhea in this case is:

a) mucosal injury by a parasite
b) osmotic effect
c) endotoxin production
d) exotoxin production
e) invasion of the mucosa for malignant cells

Items 63-64

A 65-year-old black male, heavy smoker was seen in the hospital for shortness of breath and hemoptysis. A chest-x-ray shows a 3 cm nodule in the right lung. A bronchoscopy with biopsies of the lung was performed (see figure 19).

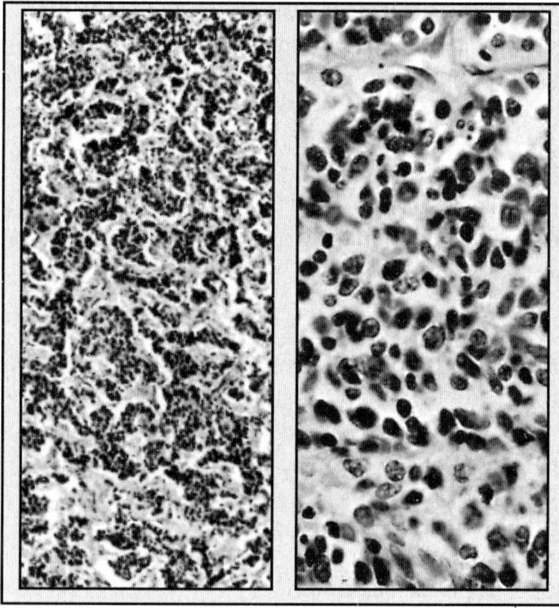

Figure 19 (Question 3.63)

63. Other manifestation(s) of this lung disease, include(s):

a) inappropriate secretion of anti-diuretic hormone
b) hypercalcemia
c) acromegaly
d) Myasthenia Gravis-like syndrome
e) all of the above

64. The most likely diagnosis in this patient is:

a) carcinoma of the lung
b) *mycobacterium TB*
c) asbestosis
d) sarcoidosis
e) no abnormalities are detected in the lungs

65. Each of the following are physiological characteristics of REM sleep, EXCEPT:

a) hyperventilation
b) increased skeletal muscle tone
c) increased heart rate
d) penile erection
e) occurrence once every 1.5 to 2 hours of sleep

66. Learned helplessness (studies in which animals are given inescapable aversive stimuli at random times) is an animal model for which of the following human disorders?

a) Major depression
b) Dependent personality disorder
c) Antisocial personality disorder
d) Conversion disorder
e) Schizophrenia

67. Which of the following muscles in the anterior fascial compartment of the forearm may be absent in healthy individuals?

a) Pronator teres
b) Pronator quadratus
c) Anconeus
d) Palmaris longus
e) Flexor carpi ulnaris

68. A man dying of cancer has severe pain which is relieved only by high doses of morphine. The concurrent deep sedation and respiratory depression hasten the man's death. Because the dying man's wishes (of pain relief) were placed first, which ethical principle was involved in the decision to administer the medication?

a) Consequentialism
b) Double Effect
c) Utilitarianism
d) Deontology
e) Teleology

69. The smooth muscle:

a) has relatively more troponin than skeletal muscle
b) contracts with less force than skeletal muscle
c) has a resting membrane potential which is less negative, and a resistance which is greater than skeletal muscle
d) contains more myosin, but less actin and tropomyosin than skeletal muscle
e) like skeletal muscle, needs ATPase activity for the formation of an inactive complex of actin/myosin

70. The septum transversum is involved in the development of:

a) cardiac chambers
b) genitourinary system
c) diaphragm muscle
d) the nose and oral palate
e) rectum

71. Which of the following may be a side-effect of physiostigmine administration?

a) Excessive salivation
b) Tachycardia
c) Constipation
d) Mydriasis
e) Urinary retention

72. Which of the following statements is true concerning nifedipine?

a) It antagonizes calcium channels
b) It is a potent diuretic
c) It is an angiotensin converting enzyme inhibitor
d) It is a first-line drug in the treatment of congestive heart failure
e) A common side effect is an increase in total peripheral resistance

73. Which of the following statements best describes the relationship between plasma cortisol and psychiatric illness?

a) Plasma cortisol is elevated in delirium
b) Plasma cortisol is elevated in depression
c) Plasma cortisol is decreased in depression
d) Plasma cortisol is elevated in anxiety disorder
e) Plasma cortisol is decreased in anxiety disorder

Items 74-75

74. Which of the following red blood cell (RBC) indices is determined by dividing the volume of packed RBCs by the RBC count?

a) Mean cell volume (MCV)
b) Mean cell hemoglobin content (MCH)
c) Mean cell hemoglobin concentration (MCHC)
d) Hematocrit (Hct)
e) Hemoglobin concentration ([Hb])

75. The hematocrit is measured in which of the following units?

a) Grams (g)
b) Grams per deciliter (g/dL)
c) Cubic micrometers (μm3)
d) Number of RBC per microliter (#RBC/μL)
e) Percent (%)

76. Which of the following muscles extends and laterally rotates the thigh at the hip?

a) Gluteus maximus
b) Gluteus medius
c) Gluteus minimus
d) Gracilis
e) Piriformis

77. Intravenous injection of sodium amobarbitol is most likely to produce which of the following?

a) Improvement in patients with dementia but not delirium
b) Improvement in patients with delirium but not dementia
c) Improvement in patients with conversion disorder
d) Increased impairment of psychotic patients
e) Increased likelihood of receiving truthful answers from an individual with antisocial personality disorder

78. Which of the following coronary arteries is most commonly occluded in patients having a myocardial infarction?

a) Marginal branch of the right coronary artery.
b) Right coronary artery near the origin.
c) Coronary sinus.
d) Circumflex branch of the left coronary artery.
e) Anterior descending branch of the left coronary artery.

Items 79-81

Match the following with the most appropriate receptor.

a) α_1 adrenergic receptor
b) ∂_2 adrenergic receptor
c) $ß_1$ adrenergic receptor
d) $ß_2$ adrenergic receptor
e) $ß_1ß_2$ adrenergic receptor

79. Metoprolol.

80. Yohimbine.

81. Isoproterenol.

82. The Wisconsin Card Sorting Test (WCST) assesses a subject's ability to shift conceptual orientations by recognizing changing patterns (shape, color, number, etc.) in a matching series of cards. As such, this test might be useful in identifying lesions in which part of the brain?

a) Prefrontal cortex
b) Parietal cortex
c) Temporal cortex
d) Occipital cortex
e) Limbic lobe

83. Each of the following statements is true of erythropoiesis, EXCEPT:

a) the spleen produces RBCs prenatally, and destroys old RBCs postnatally.
b) the liver is the primary source of RBCs for the fetus in the second trimester.
c) the medullary cavity in the ribs contributes to erythropoiesis throughout adult life.
d) the long bones (femur, tibia) are the primary source of RBCs throughout adult life.
e) erythropoietin (EPO) is the major growth factor responsible for producing RBCs and is produced in the kidney.

84. A man with portal hypertension is observed to have caput medusae (prominent veins around the umbilicus.) This is due to increased blood flow between the paraumbilical veins and:

a) the gastric veins
b) the azygous vein
c) the superior rectal vein
d) the iliac veins
e) the hepatic veins

85. Neuroimaging studies have most consistently revealed which of the following abnormalities in patients with obsessive-compulsive disorder (OCD)?

a) Enlarged lateral ventricles
b) Wide cortical sulci
c) Hypoplastic cerebellar vermis lobules
d) Increased glucose utilization in the temporal cortices
e) Reduced size of the caudate nuclei

Items 86-88

The following graph (see figure 20) depicts hormonal levels in arbitrary units, during one month of the female reproductive cycle.

Option «E» represents none of the above.

Which letter BEST represents the pattern of:

86. Luteinizing hormone.

87. Progesterone.

88. Human chorionic gonadotropin.

89. Alzheimer's dementia involves many affective and cognitive changes. Place the following changes in the temporal order in which they most typically occur, from the earliest to the latest.

1 = decreased interest, apathy, and mood changes.
2 = decline in bowel and bladder control.
3 = decline in language skills.
4 = subtle personality changes.
5 = decline in intellectual skills and memory.

a) 1 , 4 , 3 , 5 , 2
b) 4 , 1 , 5 , 3 , 2
c) 5 , 4 , 1 , 2 , 3
d) 4 , 5 , 3 , 1 , 2
e) 5 , 3 , 4 , 1 , 2

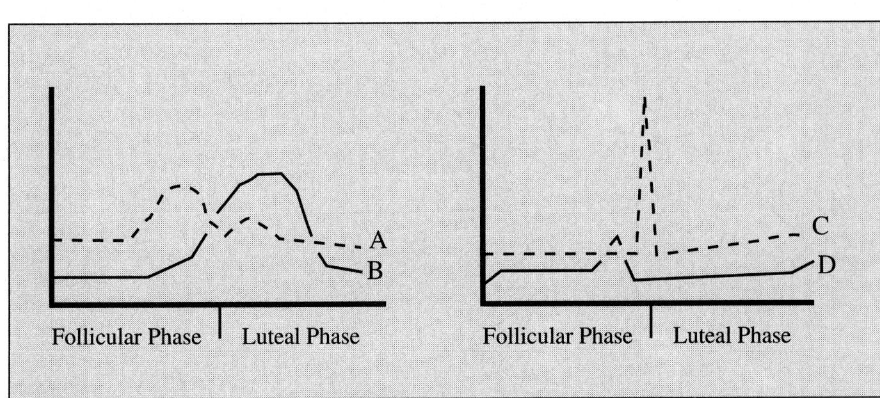

Figure 20 (Question 3.86)

90. Place the following steps of the extrinsic coagulation cascade and final common pathway in the proper sequence.

1 = thrombinogen to thrombin
2 = factor X to factor Xa
3 = factor VII to factor VIIa
4 = factor XII to factor XIIa
5 = fibrinogen to fibrin

a) 3 , 2 , 1 , 5
b) 4 , 2 , 3 , 1 , 5
c) 4 , 3 , 5 , 1
d) 3 , 1 , 2 , 4 , 5
e) 2 , 3 , 1 , 4 , 5

USMLE step 1

BASIC MEDICAL SCIENCES

BOOK F TEST 4

Questions: 90 Time: 90 minutes

1. Each of the following correctly matches a human proto-oncogene with its cellular function, EXCEPT:

	Proto-oncogene	Function
a)	*abl*	protein kinase
b)	*erb A*	steroid receptor
c)	*myc*	DNA binding protein
d)	*sis*	retinoic acid receptor
e)	*N-ras*	GTPase

2. Which of the following macromolecular interactions acts over the greatest distance?

a) Hydrogen bond
b) Dipole-dipole
c) Charge-induced dipole
d) Dipole-induced dipole
e) Dispersion

3. What is the pH of a 1M solution of lactic acid (pKa = 3.86) in which the conjugate base is ten times more concentrated than the acid?

a) 2.86
b) 3.76
c) 3.86
d) 3.96
e) 4.86

4. The diagram (see figure 21) shows the titration of a neutral amino acid with sodium hydroxide (NaOH). Which point of the curve represents the isoelectric point (pI)?

Figure 21 (Question 4.4)

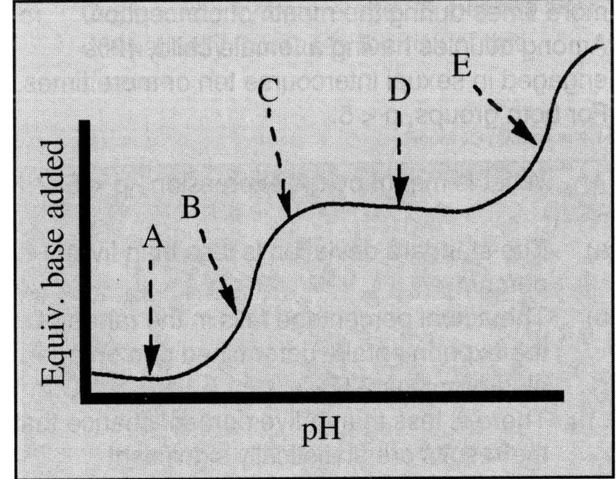

16. What is the energy charge of a cell with [ATP] = 2 mmol, [ADP] = 4 mmol, and [AMP] = 2 mmol?

a) 0.1
b) 0.25
c) 0.5
d) 0.75
e) 0.8

17. In yeast, G_1 cyclins are important for:

a) sporulation.
b) reversion to an earlier developmental state.
c) inducing apoptosis.
d) cell division.
e) transcription of genes which enable the fermentation of maltose.

18. Incorporation of which of the following amino acids is most likely to cause a deviation from the regular three-dimensional structure of a polypeptide?

a) Tryptophan
b) Cysteine
c) Lysine
d) Valine
e) Proline

19. Which of the following statements is TRUE of amino acids?

a) Phenylalanine has three ionizable subgroups
b) Most proteins absorb UV light with a peak at 180 nm
c) Lysine and arginine tend to be proton donors with regard to hydrogen bonding
d) The side group on histidine is ionized at a higher pH than is the side group on tyrosine
e) The molecular weight of leucine is less than that of lysine

20. Each of the following statements regarding peptide bonds are correct, EXCEPT:

a) the peptide bond is thermodynamically stable in an aqueous environment.
b) peptide bond synthesis is coupled to ATP hydrolysis.
c) the peptide bond is planar and cannot rotate freely.
d) trypsin cleaves to the carboxyl side of Lys or Arg.
e) chymotrypsin cleaves bonds which follow aromatic or bulky aliphatic side chains.

21. In a particular licensing examination, the mean score is 72 and the standard deviation (S.D.) is 9.0. Approximately what percentage of applicants will have scored higher than 90?

a) 0.5 %
b) 2.5 %
c) 5%
d) 10 %
e) 15 %

22. A 30 year-old white male is referred to a psychiatry for his catatonic behavior. He has a brother with schizophrenia. He is distant and isolated. He recently lost his job. He has a poor personal grooming. During the history the psychiatrist noticed his affect was flat with delusions and marked loosening of associations. This condition has been present for 2 weeks. Which of the following findings in this patient is NOT typical for schizophrenia?

a) Flat affect and poor personal grooming
b) Genetic factors have a strong influence in its development
c) Psychotic symptoms, deterioration from previous levels of functioning for less than 4 weeks
d) Flat or grossly inappropriate affect
e) It is common at teenager and/or before third decade of life

23. Which of the following sleep stages is more likely to have an episode of night terrors?

a) REM
b) NREM stage 1
c) NREM stage 2
d) NREM stage 4
e) Wakefulness

24. A 60-year-old black male was recently diagnosed with lung cancer. As a physician you may discuss the stages in the dying process as described by Kubler-Ross. You briefly may describe this process, that consists of the following stages, EXCEPT:

a) anxiety
b) bargaining
c) anger
d) acceptance
e) depression

25. In Public Health you have studied that regarding childbirth and infancy:

a) the rate of cesarean birth has decreased over the last three decades, largely due to the advent of epidural anesthesia
b) prematurity is defined as gestation of less than 34 weeks or birth weight under 2500 g
c) postpartum psychosis affects up to 0.5-1% of women after childbirth
d) the United States has the world's second-lowest rate of infant mortality
e) simple reflexes (such as the Babinski and Moro) begin to develop approximately 4 weeks after birth.

Items 26

A 34 year-old white female is seen for epistaxis and easy bruising and bleeding. At the time of admission a serum was obtained for ANA test. A picture of this test is shown in figure 24. This immunofluorescence pattern can be found in:

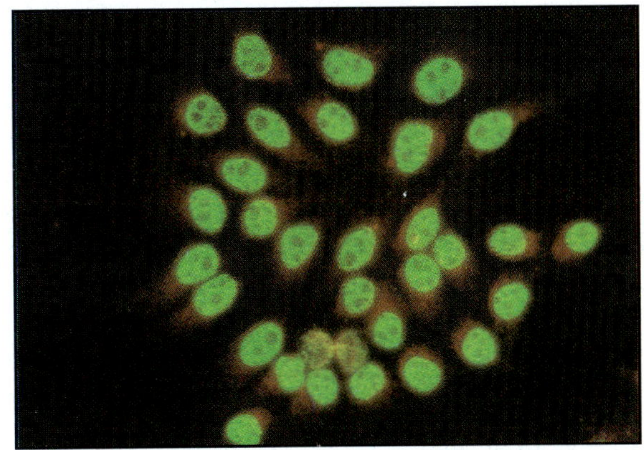

Figure 24 (Question 4.26)

a) Scleroderma
b) Rheumatoid arthritis
c) collagen vascular diseases
d) Sjogren disease
e) all of the above

Item 27-29

A 17 year-old white female is seen for abdominal pain and distention. After abdominal laparotomy was performed, an enlarged mesenteric lymph node was removed. The biopsy of this case is shown in the figure 25.

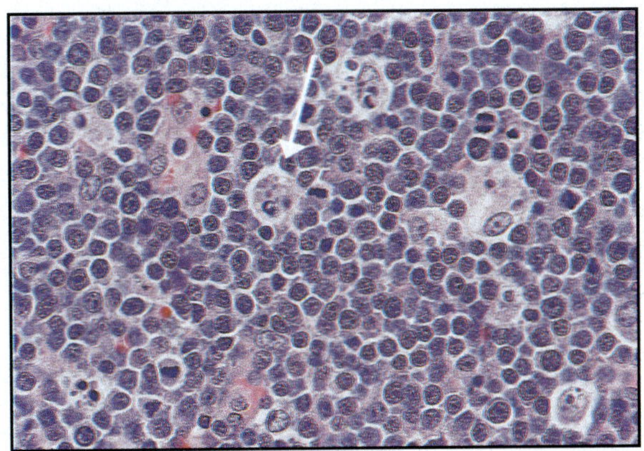

Figure 25 (Question 4.27)

27. The arrow shows:

a) a lymphocytic cell
b) a granuloma
c) a macrophage
d) a vessel
e) a muscle cell

28. The microscopic findings are most likely compatible with the diagnosis of:

a) normal tissue
b) hairy cell leukemia
c) Burkitt's lymphoma
d) sarcoma of soft tissues
e) mesothelioma

29. The characteristics of this clinical picture are the following, EXCEPT:

a) the Epstein-Barr viral genome is present in 95% of the cases in the Endemic (African) Burkitt
b) the most common sites of involvement include the jaw bones in the AIDS patients
c) 50% long-term survival with the present methods of treatment
d) most common lymphoma in AIDS patients
e) a «starry sky» appearance

Items 30-32

A 49 year-old white female was brought to the emergency room hypotensive, and comatose, after an overdose caused by a mixture of acetaminophen, aspirin and benzodiazepines. She is being assisted with a mechanical ventilator. The blood tests show:

Na	146 mEq/L	(136-145)
K	4.0 mEq/L	(3.5-5.0)
Mg	2.9 mg/dL	(1.5-2.0)
Creatinine	1.0 mg/dL	(0.6-1.2)
Glucose	116 mEq/dL	(70-120)
AST	126 mg/dL	(8-25)
ALT	646 mg/dL	(8-20)
GGTP	1146 mg/dL	(20-40)

A biopsy of the liver was performed (see figure 26).

30. The findings in the liver biopsy are the following, EXCEPT:

a) granulomatosis around the central vein
b) hepatic necrosis which is more evident around the central vein
c) hemorrhage and diffuse massive inflammatory infiltrate
d) massive inflammatory infiltrate around the central vein
e) infiltration of malignant cells around the central vein

31. One useful medical treatment in this patient may include:

a) acetylcysteine
b) morphine
c) high doses of steroids
d) gancyclovir
e) methanol

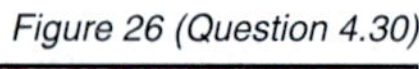
Figure 26 (Question 4.30)

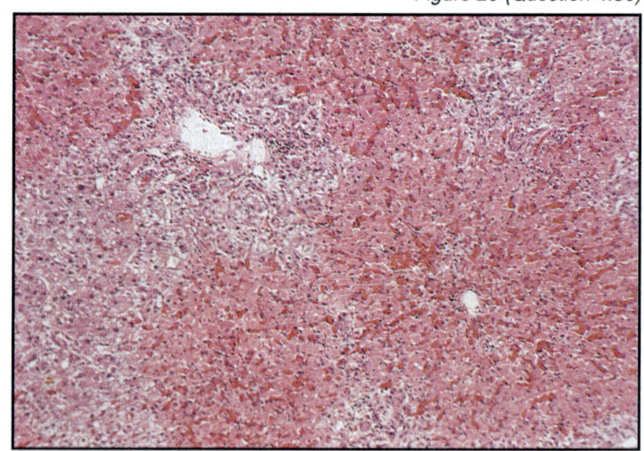

32. The most likely liver toxicity in this patient is caused by:

a) aspirin
b) benzodiazepines
c) hypotension
d) acetaminophen
e) liver histopathology is normal

33. The following sequence is a synthetic mRNA, including start and stop signals.

5' ... CGCTAGAUGUCCTCUAACTUAGCCUAGTGGUGATTT ... 3'

This mRNA encodes an oligopeptide of:

a) three residues
b) six residues
c) nine residues
d) ten residues
e) twelve residues

34. What is the correct sequence of events in the synthesis of insulin?

1=cleavage of C peptide
2=leader sequence cleaved
3=polypeptide in random coil form
4=disulfide bonds formed
5=polypeptide located in secretory granule

a) 2, 3, 4, 5, 1
b) 3, 2, 1, 5, 4
c) 5, 3, 2, 4, 1
d) 5, 2, 3, 4, 1
e) 3, 2, 4, 1, 5

35. Each of the following effects favors the folding of a globular protein, EXCEPT:

a) an increase in the number of internal hydrogen bonds between amino acids
b) placing hydrophobic amino acids on the inside of the molecule
c) decreasing the entropy of the protein
d) making the enthalpy of the folding reaction more negative
e) electrostatic interaction between amino acid side chains

36. In operant conditioning:

a) a behavior is emitted in anticipation of a reinforcer
b) a reinforcer precedes and induces a behavior
c) a stimulus induces a reflexive response
d) a reflex happens in anticipation of a stimulus
e) an aversive stimulus is positively reinforced

37. A twelve month-old child can speak a few simple words, and can stand but not walk. Which of the following is true regarding this pattern of development?

	Speech development	Motor development
a)	Delayed	Delayed
b)	Normal	Delayed
c)	Delayed	Normal
d)	Accelerated	Delayed
e)	Normal	Normal

38. On an electroencephalogram (EEG), which of the following wave types would be seen during attentiveness with eyes open?

a) alpha
b) beta
c) gamma
d) delta
e) theta

39. The mini-mental state test directly assesses each of the following parameters, EXCEPT:

a) orientation
b) calculation
c) ability to copy an object
d) abstract reasoning
e) recall

Items 40-41

Choose the appropriate diagnosis from the list below.

a) Schizoid personality disorder
b) Schizotypal personality disorder
c) Antisocial personality disorder
d) Avoidant personality disorder
e) Borderline personality disorder

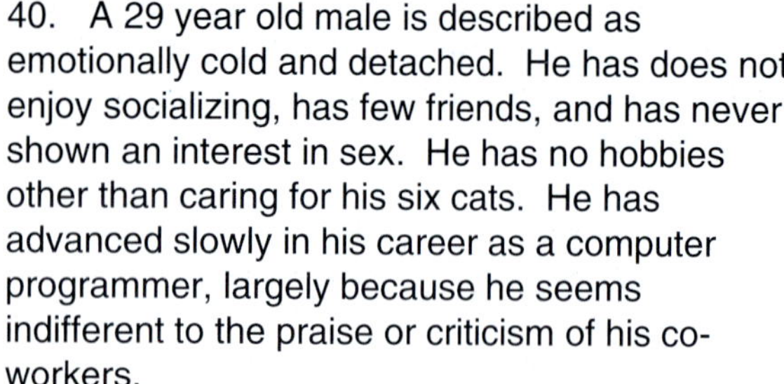

40. A 29 year old male is described as emotionally cold and detached. He has does not enjoy socializing, has few friends, and has never shown an interest in sex. He has no hobbies other than caring for his six cats. He has advanced slowly in his career as a computer programmer, largely because he seems indifferent to the praise or criticism of his co-workers.

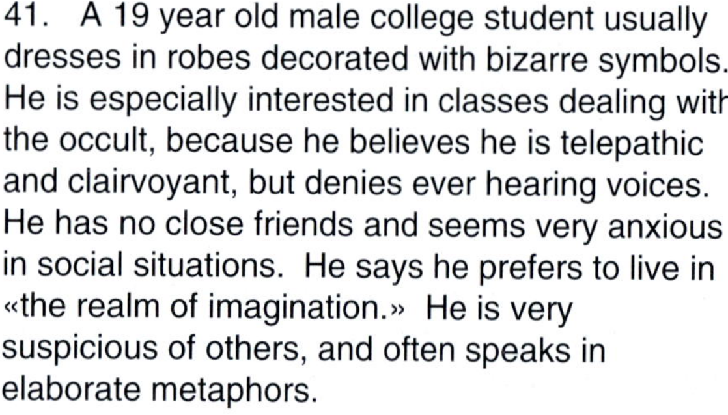

41. A 19 year old male college student usually dresses in robes decorated with bizarre symbols. He is especially interested in classes dealing with the occult, because he believes he is telepathic and clairvoyant, but denies ever hearing voices. He has no close friends and seems very anxious in social situations. He says he prefers to live in «the realm of imagination.» He is very suspicious of others, and often speaks in elaborate metaphors.

Items 42-44

A 34 year-old white female comes to the medical office for her annual check-up. A PAP smear was performed (see figure 27)

42. The presence of these cells in the PAP smear is MOST likely to represent:

a) a normal PAP smear
b) carcinoma of the endocervix
c) colonization of the endocervix by *Trichomonas vaginalis*
d) a yeast infection of the vaginal mucosa
e) atypical endocervical cells of undetermined significance

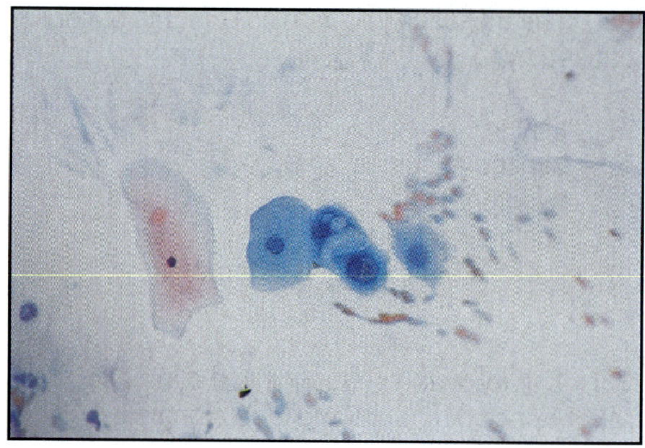

Figure 27 (Question 4.42)

43. The histological findings in this PAP smear, suggest that this female probably has been exposed to:

a) Human Papilloma Virus (HPV)
b) Human Immunodeficiency Virus (HIV)
c) estrogens exogenous
d) gonorrhea
e) syphilis

44. The following statements regarding her histological findings are correct, EXCEPT:

a) adenocarcinoma of the endocervix accounts for 10% of malignant cervical tumors
b) the mean age at presentation of this clinical condition is 56 years of age
c) it is associated to adenocarcinoma in situ
d) squamous cell carcinoma is typical of this condition with cytoplasmatic vacuolation
e) they represent a life-threatening illness

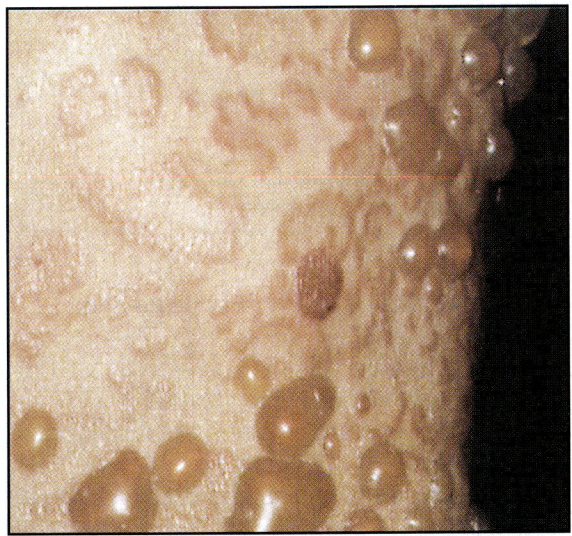

Figure 28a (Question 4.45)

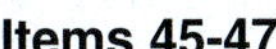

Items 45-47

A 50-year-old white male presents several skin lesions as seen in the figure 28a. A skin biopsy was obtained and the tissue was stained with goat-fluorescinated anti-human IgG (green stain in the figure 28b).

45. The most likely diagnosis is:

a) Acanthosis Nigricans
b) Pemphigus Vulgaris
c) basal cell carcinoma
d) skin abscess
e) melanoma

46. The most likely etiology of this condition is:

a) infectious
b) neoplastic
c) autoimmune
d) hereditary
e) traumatic

47. Most likely, the structures stained by the goat-fluorescinated anti-human IgG are:

a) the cytoplasm
b) the desmosomes
c) the mitochondria
d) the cell nuclei
e) the epidermal connective tissue

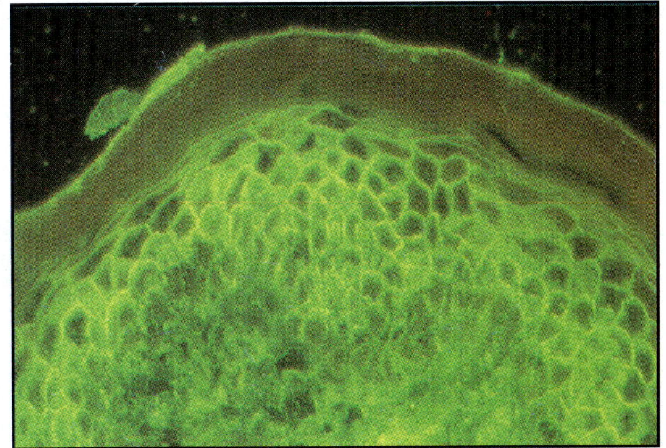

Figure 28b (Question 4.45)

48. The immunoglobulin variable domain is oriented into a barrel of antiparallel ß pleated sheets. This is an example of:

a) primary protein structure
b) secondary protein structure
c) tertiary protein structure
d) quaternary protein structure
e) none of the above

49. The enzyme pyruvate carboxylase is:

a) an isomerase
b) a transferase
c) a ligase
d) a lyase
e) a hydrolase

50. Which of the following statements is true of enzyme inhibition?

a) A noncompetitive inhibitor binds covalently at the active site.
b) A competitive inhibitor increases the Vmax.
c) A competitive inhibitor decreases the K_M.
d) A noncompetitive inhibitor decreases the Vmax.
e) A competitive inhibitor binds covalently at the active site.

51. Trypsin and chymotrypsin are proteases that have which of the following amino acid residues at their active sites?

a) Alanine
b) Cysteine
c) Glutamic acid
d) Serine
e) Threonine

52. The intracellular trafficking of protein G is analyzed using subcellular fractionation in a density gradient. At a particular time point, radio-labelled protein G is found to be associated with a fraction positive for α-mannosidase. This fraction most likely represents which of the following organelles?

a) Golgi apparatus
b) Rough endoplasmic reticulum (RER)
c) Nucleus
d) Mitochondria
e) Lysosome

Items 53-55

A 24 year-old white male is admitted to the ICU for acute renal failure and hemoptysis (coughing bright red blood). His urinalysis also showed macrohematuria (blood in urine). The chest-x-ray showed infiltration in several lung lobes. A biopsy of the right kidney with immunostaining of the glomeruli was obtained (see figure 29).

Figure 29 (Question 4.53)

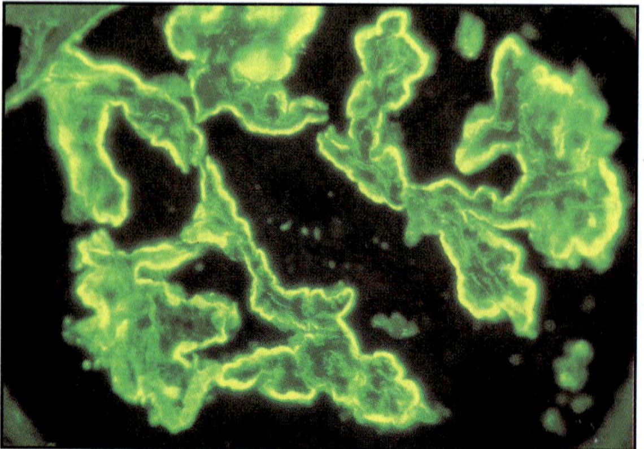

53. The most likely diagnosis is:

a) Tuberculosis
b) Nephrolithiasis
c) Nephrotic syndrome
d) Acute ischemic tubular necrosis
e) Goodpasture syndrome

54. The histopathological findings are the following, EXCEPT:

a) bacterial infiltrate in the nephron
b) anti-glomerular-membrane basal staining in the kidney
c) anti-glomerular-membrane basal staining in the lung
d) inflammatory exudative process in the lung
e) an immune-inflammatory process in the lung

55. The MOST typical feature of this disease is:

a) the presence of anti-cytoplasmatic antibodies
b) the presence of anti-basement membrane antibodies
c) the presence of anti-native DNA antibodies
d) the presence of anti-mitochondrial antibodies
e) none of the above

Figure 30 (Question 4.56)

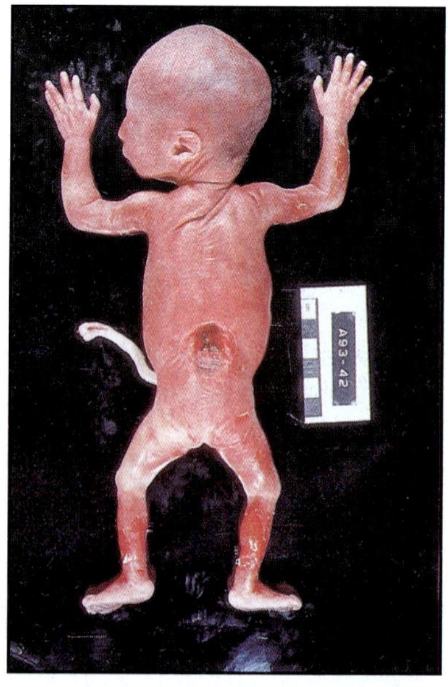

Items 56-57

The figure 30 shows a newborn who died few hours after delivery.

56. The most likely diagnosis is:

a) Microcephalus
b) Abscess in the spinal axis
c) Arnold Chiari malformation
d) Anencephaly
e) Down syndrome

57. Other most common brain stem and cerebellum abnormalities associated to this syndrome are the following, EXCEPT:

a) displacement of the cerebellar tonsils into the cervical canal
b) Z kink distortion of the medulla at the cervicomedullary junction
c) a small, shallow posterior fossa with enlarged foramen magnum
d) hydrocephalus and spinal dysraphism
e) cerebellar oligoganglioma

Items 58-59

A 40 year-old white male with a history of heavy smoking is concerned that he may have lung cancer. The medical resident ordered a cytology of the sputum which is shown in the figure 31.

58. The most likely histological findings in this picture is:

a) inflammatory cells suggesting acute bronchitis
b) malignant cells, suggesting neoplastic tumor
c) normal bronchial epithelial cells
d) asbestos bodies in the sputum
e) bronchial epithelium infested with *Mycobacterium TB*

59. This sputum sample is:

a) suboptimal for analysis because of bronchial contaminants
b) only appropriate for the analysis of the oral cavity pathology, because the presence of saliva elements
c) optimal for analysis because the presence bronchial epithelial cells
d) optimal for analysis because of the presence of macrophages without bronchial epithelium
e) none of the above is correct

Figure 31 (Question 4.58)

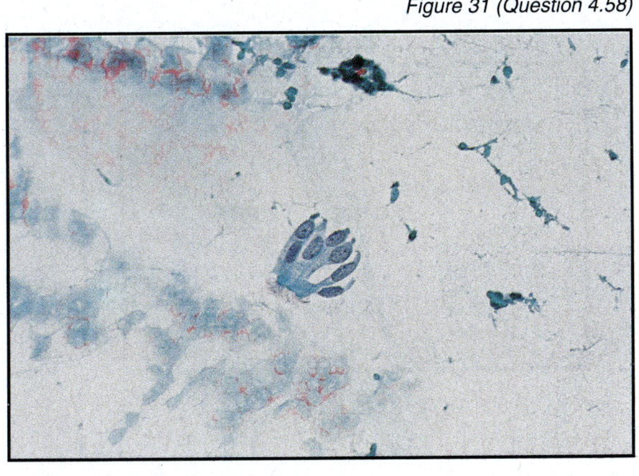

Figure 32 (Question 4.60)

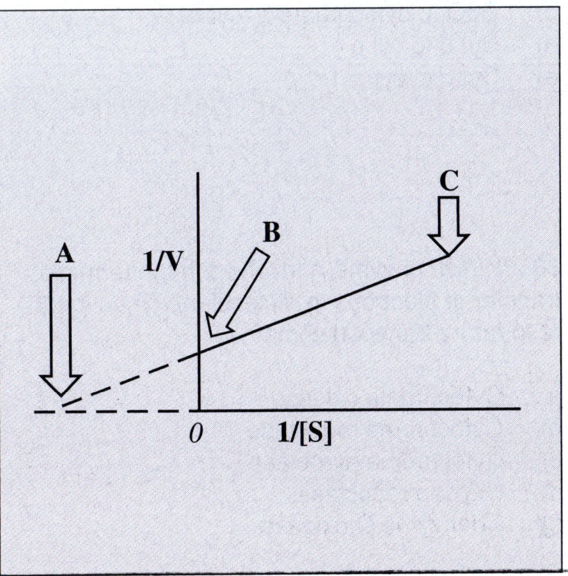

Items 60-61

Use the following choices to answer the questions pertaining to the Lineweaver-Burke plot generated using data from an enzyme kinetics experiment. (see figure 32).

(V = reaction velocity,. [S] = substrate concentration.)

a) A
b) 1/A
c) A/2
d) B
e) 1/B

60. Which is the maximal reaction velocity obtainable in this experiment?

61. What is the negative reciprocal of the Michaelis constant, K_M, for the enzyme in the reaction?

62. Which of the following electron transfers between respiratory electron carriers at the inner mitochondrial membrane involves the largest absolute change in standard reduction potential, and hence might be coupled to ATP synthesis?

a) NADH to Flavin mononucleotide (FMN)
b) FMN to Coenzyme Q (CoQ)
c) CoQ to cytochrome b (cyt b)
d) Cyt b to cyt a
e) Cyt c to cyt a

63. Which enzyme is involved in the terminal transfer of electrons to molecular oxygen in the respiratory transport chain?

a) Cytochrome oxidase
b) Cytochrome reductase
c) Cytochrome hydrolase
d) Oxygen reductase
e) Coenzyme Q oxidase

64. If 3 NADH molecules and 2 FADH molecules enter the electron transport chain, what is the maximum number of ATP molecules that could be produced?

a) 5
b) 10
c) 11
d) 12
e) 13

65. Hemoglobin S:

a) results from a mutation at the 17th base in the ß chain
b) results from a substitution of valine for glutamate in the alpha chain
c) results from aberrant post-translational processing
d) causes erythrocytes to aggregate in oxygen-poor conditions
e) is an X-linked variant which offers a selective advantage against malaria in endemic areas

66. Figure 33 shows a gel electrophoresis (pH 8.5) run on hemoglobin samples. Which sample is most likely from a person with sickle cell disease (homozygous HbS)?

a) A
b) B
c) C
d) A or C, depending on the buffer
e) Cannot be determined

Figure 33 (Question 4.66)

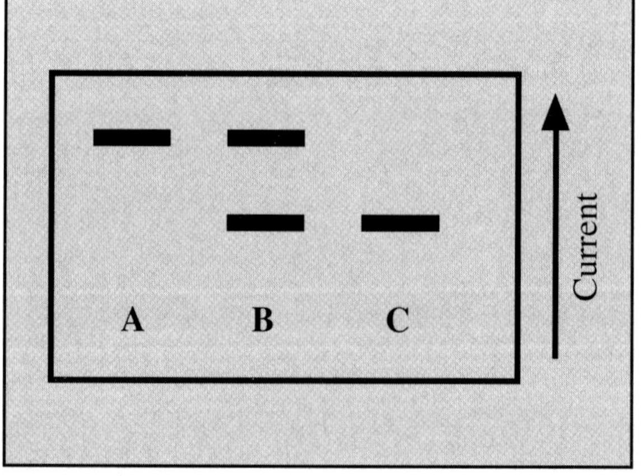

67. Which of the following is the best example of an «open-ended question»?

a) Why are you crying?
b) Can you tell me whether you've been hospitalized in the past?
c) How bad is the pain?
d) Can you tell me about the problem you've been having with your back?
e) Don't you want to get well?

68. The following conflicts represent behavioral milestones in childhood development as described by Erikson. Which sequence is placed in the proper temporal order?

1 = Autonomy vs shame and doubt.
2 = Identity vs diffusion.
3 = Industry vs inferiority.
4 = Initiative vs guilt .
5 = Trust vs mistrust.

a) 1 , 4 , 3 , 2 , 5
b) 5 , 4 , 1 , 2 , 3
c) 5 , 1 , 4 , 3 , 2
d) 5 , 4 , 3 , 1 , 2
e) 1 , 5 , 3 , 2 , 4

69. The following set of numbers represent the number of family members in a population of families exposed to high levels of electromagnetic radiation. What is the median of the set?

4, 3, 5, 4, 3, 6, 3, 6, 5

a) 3
b) 4
c) 4.3
d) 4.67
e) 5

70. People living in which of the following U.S. regions might be expected to experience the greatest barrier to health care access and delivery?

a) Pacific northwest
b) Midwest
c) New England
d) Southern Pacific coast
e) South

Items 71-73

In a clinical trial, a new pregnancy test is tried by 100 women known to be pregnant and 100 women known not to be pregnant.

I. Of those known to be pregnant, 90 test positive.
II. Of those known not to be pregnant, 30 test positive.

Choose the most appropriate answer from the following list:

a) 90%
b) 85%
c) 80%
d) 75%
e) 70%

71. What is the specificity of the test?

72. What is the sensitivity of the test?

73. What is the chance a woman testing positive will actually be pregnant?

74. After experiencing a decline in exam performance in a certain class, a medical student begins to attend fewer lectures. This may be interpreted as an example of which type of conditioning?

a) Extinction
b) Operant reflex
c) Transference
d) Habituation
e) Sensitization

75. Which type of psychological test involves asking a subject to respond to vague, ambiguous stimuli in order to gain insight into the subject's unconscious?

a) Intelligence test
b) Personality inventory
c) Projective test
d) Test for coarse brain disease
e) Holmes-Rahe life change scale

76. Which of the following nonspecific symptoms is LEAST likely to be associated with somatization disorder?

a) Shortness of breath
b) Dysmenorrhea
c) Vomiting
d) Chest pain
e) Amnesia

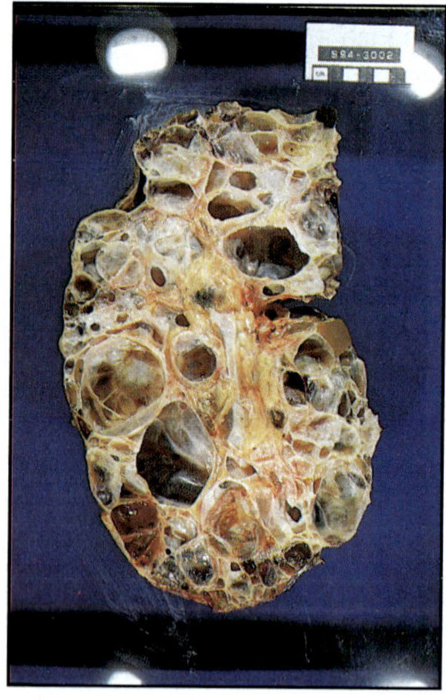

Figure 34 (Question 4.77)

Items 77-78

Figure 34 shows the kidney of a patient who died of end-stage kidney disease.

77. The MOST likely underlying disease is:

a) nephrocalcinosis
b) polycystic kidney disease
c) pyelonephritis
d) rapidly progressive proliferative glomerulonephritis
e) none of the above

78. The most common features of this disease include the following, EXCEPT:

a) it causes end-stage renal failure in at least 8% of the patients
b) it is usually originated from chronic infection of the kidney medulla
c) Fifteen percent of the patients develop a brain aneurysm
d) it is usually inherited
e) it is associated with liver cysts

Items 79-80

A 65 year-old white female presents the lesions seen in figure 35. A biopsy of the same lesions is reported as follows: « superficial perivascular, lymphocytic infiltrate with dermal edema, and margination of lymphocytes along the dermal-epidermal junction. These lymphocytes are intimately associated with degenerating and necrotic keratinocytes».

79. The most likely diagnosis of this clinical-pathological case is:

a) Measles
b) skin abscesses
c) Bullous pemphigoid
d) Erythema multiform
e) melanomas

80. This disease can be associated with:

a) side effects of sulfas
b) side effects of phenytoin
c) systemic lupus erythematous
d) lymphomas
e) all of the above

Figure 35 (Question 4.79)

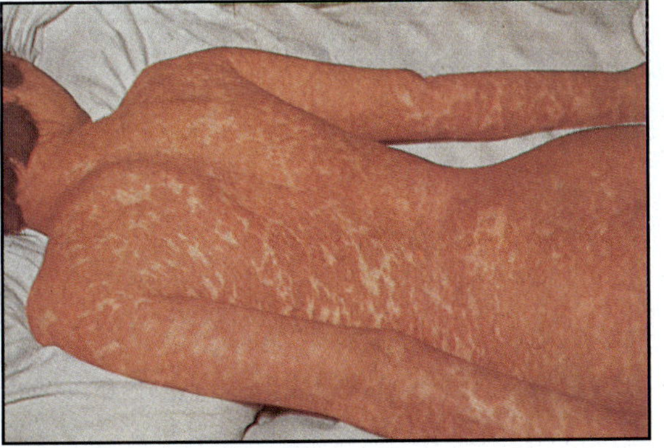

Item 81

A 22 year-old white female is seen for the presence of a supraclavicular lymph node. The lymph node is mobile and painful to the manual palpation. A biopsy of the lymph node stained with CD20 (which stains B-lymphocytes) is seen in figure 36.

81. The most likely histopathological diagnosis is:

a) T-cell lymphoma
b) B-cell lymphoma
c) Burkitt lymphoma
d) Hairy cell leukemia
e) Hyperplastic lymph nodes

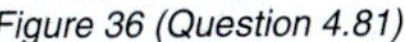

Figure 36 (Question 4.81)

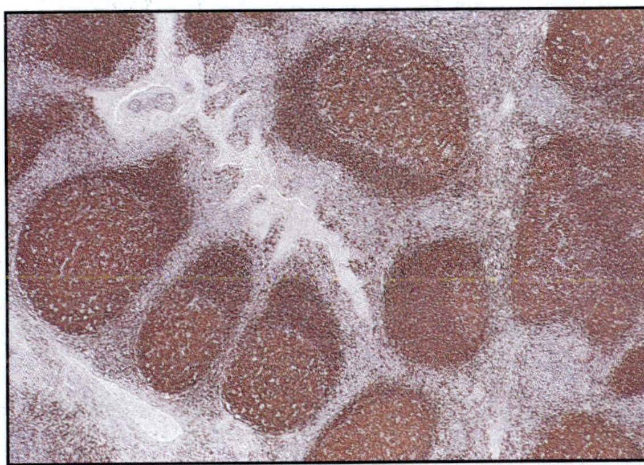

Items 82-84

A 3 year-old white boy complains of pain in his left flank for several months. He developed gross hematuria 2 days later. A mass was also palpated in the left flank. A laparostomy with left nephrectomy was performed. The biopsy of the left kidney is shown in figure 37.

82. The most likely diagnosis is:

a) hydronephrosis
b) Wilms tumor
c) pyelonephritis with abceration
d) sarcoma
e) nephrocalcinosis

83. Which of the following BEST describes the findings in this biopsy?

a) Severe inflammatory infiltrate
b) Normal glomerular epithelium
c) Highly cellular tissue with undifferentiated blastema, loose stroma and immature tubules
d) Glandular, adenomatosous formation
e) Epithelial tumor with benign appearance

Items 84-85

A 40 year-old white female presents with shortness of breath, esophageal spasm, and calcification in the skin (subcutaneous). After having several episodes of hemoptysis, a lung biopsy was obtained (see figure 38).

84. The abnormal histopathological finding(s) in this picture is (are):

a) the presence of granulomas
b) the presence of eosinophilic infiltrate in the alveolar space
c) the presence of interstitial infiltrate with fibrosis and normal vessels
d) the honey-comb pattern
e) the presence of alveolar fibrosis with fibrous thickening of the small lung vessels

85. The most likely diagnosis in this patient is:

a) sarcoidosis
b) Crest syndrome
c) lymphoma
d) lung cancer
e) pneumonia

Figure 37 (Question 4.82)

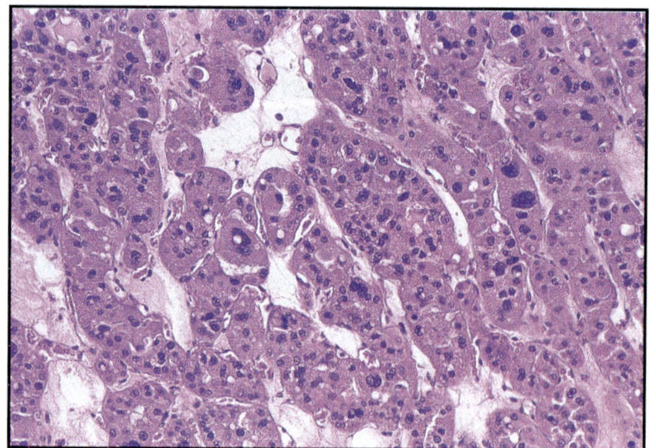

Figure 38 (Question 4.84)

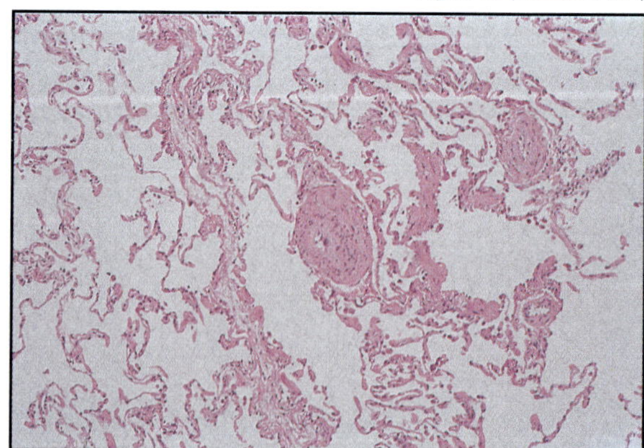

86. Which axis of the DSM IV multiaxial diagnostic system deals with psychosocial and environmental problems?

a) Axis I
b) Axis II
c) Axis III
d) Axis IV
e) Axis V

87. Which of the following statements is CORRECT regarding bipolar disorder?

a) The average age of onset is younger than that for schizophrenia
b) There is a higher than average incidence among individuals of low socioeconomic status
c) Up to 20% of the patients experience only manic episodes
d) With appropriate treatment, over 75% of patients recover completely, without recurrence
e) A good prognosis is associated with early age of onset and male gender

88. The most appropriate medical management for bipolar disorder, includes:

a) trazodone and fluoxetine
b) clozapine and valproic acid
c) chlorpromazine and amitriptyline
d) chlorpromazine and lithium
e) amitriptyline and lithium

89. Which of the following types of drugs are considered to be LEAST addicting?

a) Barbiturates
b) Alcohol
c) Tricyclic antidepressants
d) Opioids
e) Benzodiazepines

90. A certain bacterial pathogen has a high rate of infection in a given population of people. The infection is easily recognizable and readily cured with antibiotics. Even when untreated, the infection lasts only 3 weeks. However, due to the presence of numerous serotypes, people who recover from an infection are not immune from subsequent infections. Thus, for a given year:

a) the incidence is greater than prevalence
b) the prevalence is greater than incidence
c) the incidence and prevalence are equal
d) the infection rate is greater than cure rate
e) the infection rate and prevalence are equal

USMLE step 1

BASIC MEDICAL SCIENCES

BOOK F TEST 5

Questions: 90 Time: 90 minutes

1. Which of the following viruses might be most useful in carrying trophic factors into damaged neurons to improve the regeneration process?

a) Adenovirus
b) Herpes simplex virus
c) Human immunodeficiency virus (HIV)
d) Moloney murine leukemia virus
e) Vaccinia virus

2. Which one of the following relations between the cranial nerve pairs and its fibers is INCORRECT?

a) Cranial nerve III carries parasympathetic fibers
b) Cranial nerve V carries parasympathetic fibers
c) Cranial nerve VII carries parasympathetic fibers
d) Cranial nerve IX carries parasympathetic fibers
e) Cranial nerve X carries parasympathetic fibers

3. The structure shown in figure 39 most likely, represents:

a) a molecule of serum IgM
b) a molecule of serum IgA
c) a molecule of secretory IgA
d) a molecule of surface IgM
e) a molecule of surface IgD

Figure 39 (Question 5.3)

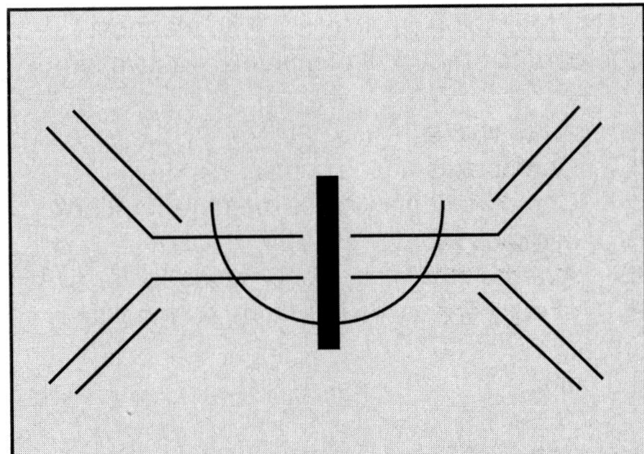

TEST 5

4. In molecular biology, some eukaryotic organisms are used as vectors and for cloning techniques. Which of the following eukaryotic microorganisms can be used as a cloning vector and a vector for expressing cloned genes?

a) *Borrelia hermsii*
b) *Saccharomyces cerevisiae*
c) *Escherishia coli*
d) *Coccidioides immitis*
e) *Actinomyces israelii*

5. The trochlear nerve (CN IV):

a) it is the smallest cranial nerve
b) it is the only nerve to exit from the dorsal aspect of the brainstem
c) it is the only nerve in which all of the lower motor neurons axons decussate
d) it has the longest intracranial course
e) all of the above

Items 6-8

Match the biological activities with the most appropriate product of complement activation.

a) Anaphylaxis
b) Chemotaxis of eosinophils
c) Component of cytolytic membrane attack complex (MAC)
d) Acted on by decay-accelerating factor (DAF)
e) directly enhances leukocyte phagocytosis

6. C5b.

7. C4a.

8. C5 convertase.

9. The following findings are correlated with the clinical progression of AIDS in a given patient, EXCEPT:

a) increased viral diversity
b) decrease in cutaneous T lymphocyte reactivity
c) increased turnover of CD4+ cells
d) increased RNA levels of HIV-1
e) dysregulation of suppressor T lymphocyte response

10. Which of the following components of the central nervous system is most likely to proliferate in response to injury?

a) Astrocytes
b) Oligodendrocytes
c) Microglia
d) Ependymal cells
e) Neurons

11. The synthesis of both DNA and proteins occurs as a unidirectional process. Which of the following statements regarding this process is CORRECT?

(N = amino-terminal, C = carboxyl-terminal; 3' and 5' refer to carbon atoms on a sugar molecule on the newly-synthesized strand).

	Direction of protein synthesis	**Direction of DNA synthesis**
a)	C –> N	3' –> 5'
b)	N –> C	3' –> 5'
c)	C –> N	5' –> 3'
d)	N –> C	5 '–> 3'
e)	None of above	

12. Which of the following best describes the relative abundances of the three types of ribonucleic acids in the cells?

M = messenger RNA;
R = ribosomal RNA;
T = transfer RNA

a) R > T > M
b) M > T > R
c) T > R > M
d) M > R > T
e) R > M > T

13. In a particular licensing examination, the mean score is 72 and the standard deviation is 9.0. Approximately what percentage of applicants will have scored higher than 90?

a) 0.5%
b) 2.5%
c) 5%
d) 10%
e) 15%

14. Schizophrenia:

a) has a 6% lifetime risk of developing
b) has strong genetic factors
c) has a prevalence equal between ages
d) is classified as a mood disorder and is best treated with a heterocyclic antidepressant
e) seldom develops prior to the age of 35

15. A 34 year-old white male with a history of acute leukemia in remission presents with fever. He has a pus-draining intravenous line, placed in his subclavian vein for chemiotherapy treatment. A culture of the catheter grew a *S. aureus* methicillin-resistant. Which of the following is the antibiotic of choice to treat this infection?

a) Vancomycin
b) Clindamycin
c) Cloxacillin
d) Third generation cephalosporins
e) Aminoglycosides

16. Which of the following apolipoproteins are found on chylomicrons but not on high-density lipoproteins (HDL)?

a) Apo A-1
b) Apo B-48
c) Apo C-1
d) Apo C-2
e) Apo D

Items 17 - 19

Match the arachidonic acid pathways with its MOST likely features

a) Cyclooxygenase (CO) pathway
b) Lipoxygenase (LO) pathway
c) Both CO and LO pathways
d) Phospholipase A_2 pathway
e) All of the above

17. Pathway(s) which lead(s) to leukotriene B_4 (LTB_4) production.

18. Pathway(s) which lead(s) to thromboxane production.

19. Pathway(s) which are significantly targeted by aspirin and indomethacin.

Items 20-22

Match the type of leukocyte with its MOST likely function or structure.

a) Basophil
b) Eosinophil
c) Lymphocyte
d) Monocyte
e) Neutrophil

20. Specific granules have a dense core (crystalloid) of cytotoxic basic proteins.

21. Granular contents are released upon binding the Fc region of IgE.

22. A small nuclear appendage («drumstick») is visible on these cells of female subjects.

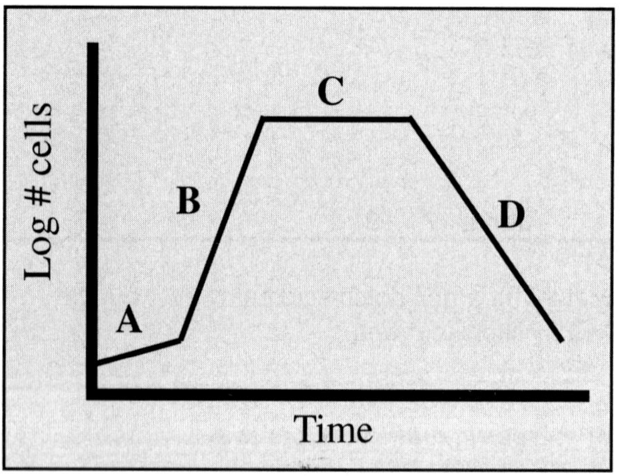

Figure 40 (Question 5.23)

23. A bacterial colony was placed in nutrient media then agitated in a 37°C incubator for several hours. Which point on the growth curve seen in the figure 40 represents the lag phase? («E» = «not shown.»)

24. Each of the following symptoms is characteristic of Kluver-Bucy syndrome EXCEPT:

a) absence of emotional responses such as fear and aggression
b) compulsive attentiveness to objects (orality)
c) hypersexuality
d) loss of recent memory
e) visual agnosia

25. The following statements regarding the surface glycoproteins on lymphocytes are correct, EXCEPT:

a) CD40 is found on the surface of T cells and is a co-stimulator for T cell activation
b) CD28 is a found on the surface of T cells and is a co-stimulator for T cell activation
c) CD3 is a signal transducing element of the T cell receptor
d) CD2 is present on T cells and has an affinity for sheep red blood cells
e) the CD45 RO marker is found on memory T cells

26. What is the most common genus associated with bacterial meningitis in each of the following age groups?

	Infants	Children	Adults
a)	Escherichia	Streptococcus	Hemophilus
b)	Staphylococcus	Listeria	Neisseria
c)	Neisseria	Hemophilus	Listeria
d)	Streptococcus	Hemophilus	Streptococcus
e)	Hemophilus	Neisseria	Staphylococcus

27. Which one of the following statements regarding the cerebral hemisphere dominant for language expression is CORRECT?

a) It is usually the right hemisphere in right-handed individuals and the left hemisphere in left-handed individuals
b) It is usually the left hemisphere in right-handed individuals and the right hemisphere in left-handed individuals
c) It is usually the right hemisphere, regardless of handedness
d) It is usually the left hemisphere, regardless of handedness
e) It is usually the left hemisphere in males and the right hemisphere in females

Items 28-29

Choose the most appropriate Streptococcal organism in each of the following scenarios.

a) *S. agalactiae*
b) *S. faecalis*
c) *S. pneumoniae*
d) *S. pyogenes*
e) *S. viridans*

28. Alpha hemolytic, resistant to optochin.

29. Beta hemolytic, sensitive to bacitracin.

30. Mitochondrial DNA:

a) is replicated in the nucleus and transported into mitochondria by protein chaperones
b) has a lower mutation rate than nuclear DNA
c) has a high rate of recombination during replication
d) is a maternal copy or a paternal copy, but not both
e) is translated using a genetic code which differs from that used by nuclear DNA

31. The following defense mechanisms described by Kubler-Ross are present in the dying process, EXCEPT:

a) anxiety
b) bargaining
c) anger
d) acceptance
e) depression

32. During childbirth and infancy:

a) the rate of cesarean birth has decreased over the last three decades, largely due to the advent of epidural anesthesia
b) prematurity is defined as gestation of less than 34 weeks or birth weight under 2500 g
c) postpartum psychosis affects up to 0.5-1% of women after childbirth
d) the United States has the world's second-lowest rate of infant mortality
e) simple reflexes (such as the Babinski and Moro) begin to develop approximately 4 weeks after birth

33. The following are health-related features of people in the low socioeconomic status, EXCEPT:

a) greater chance of self-medicating or seeing nonmedical personnel for treatment.
b) greater incidence of mental illness.
c) lower chance of eating a balanced diet.
d) greater differentiation of gender roles.
e) shorter hospital stay and relatively less sick when admitted.

Items 34-35

Match the most appropriate personality disorder for the patient condition described.

a) Borderline
b) Histrionic
c) Dependent
d) Narcissistic
e) Obsessive-compulsive

34. Despite making very slow progress toward his degree, a 32 year-old graduate student, loves to talk about his intelligence and achievements. He is very arrogant, and believes others are envious of his «special talents.» He often talks about the success and power he'll have when his «brilliance is finally recognized.»

35. A 30 year-old secretary always seems to be the center of attention. She is very theatrical and tends to exaggerate everything. Her emotions shift rapidly from laughter to tears. She dresses in a provocative manner, and constantly flirts with her co-workers.

36. Which of the following compounds binds specifically to tyrosine residues in proteins, cross-links sulfhydryl groups in enzymes and is clinically utilized for disinfecting ?

a) Hydrogen peroxide
b) Glutaraldehyde
c) Phenol
d) Ethanol
e) Iodine

Items 37-38

37. In a particular pathway of receptor-mediated endocytosis, a receptor-ligand complex is bound and internalized. After intracellular processing, the receptor is recycled back to the membrane while the ligand is degraded. Which of the following lists the MOST likely sequence of organelles through which the ligand is processed?

a) Lysosome, nucleus, endosome
b) Endosome, nucleus, endoplasmic reticulum, Golgi apparatus
c) Lysosome, endosome
d) Endosome, Golgi apparatus, lysosome
e) Endoplasmic reticulum, Golgi apparatus, endosome, lysosome

38. In the above ligand-receptor system, movement of the ligand from the cell-surface to internal organelles is inhibited by incubating the cells in colchicine. This occurs due to the fact that colchicine:

a) binds the receptor and acts as an allosteric regulator
b) inhibits microtubule interactions
c) activates nuclear transcription factors to increase production of a protein that rapidly degrades the ligand
d) induces apoptosis
e) is a competitive inhibitor of cyclic AMP

39. The homeobox genes are most important in:

a) limb development.
b) neural tube induction.
c) induction of excision-repair to remove damaged DNA.
d) shifting the reading frame for translating nested genes.
e) pattern formation and migration of neural crest cells.

40. The gene for elastin is closely linked to a gene involved in spatial orientation in the chromosome 7. An individual with a mutation in this chromosomal region might be expected to have:

a) absent hyaline cartilage and inability to copy a design
b) neglect of one side of the body and osteoporosis
c) inability to put together jigsaw puzzles and aortic malformations
d) hyperextensibility and intention tremor
e) fragile bones and inability to read (alexia)

41. The mammals that MOST likely are carriers of rabies are:

a) bats
b) domestic dogs
c) possums
d) mice and rats
e) deer and sheep

42. Which of the following sensations is transmitted through nerve fibers with the greatest conduction velocity?

a) Pressure
b) Fast pain
c) Slow pain
d) Warm temperature
e) Cold temperature

Items 43-45

Match the following interleukin (IL) with its MOST appropriate function.

a) IL-1
b) IL-2
c) IL-4
d) IL-5
e) IL-6

43. It mediates changes in the levels of acute phase proteins.

44. It activates helper and cytotoxic T cells.

45. It is required for antibody class switch and enhances synthesis of IgE.

Items 46-48

Choose the most likely diagnosis in each of the following cases of atypical pneumonia.

a) *Chlamydial pneumonia*
b) *Influenza*
c) *Legionnaires' disease*
d) *Mycoplasmal pneumonia*
e) *Q fever*

46. An 18 year-old female college student experienced the gradual onset of a nonproductive cough and sore throat. Chest X-ray shows patchy hilar infiltrates. Laboratory findings include antibodies to red blood cells (cold agglutinins). Her condition improves after taking erythromycin.

47. A 49 year-old male cattle farmer experiences the rapid onset of fever, headache, and coughing. Chest X-ray shows a patchy infiltrate, and liver function tests are abnormal.

48. During the summer, a 58 year-old woman experiences a severe cough with confusion and diarrhea. Urinalysis shows proteinuria, and a sputum stain shows faint, gram-negative rods.

49. Which of the following substances is a strong polyclonal activator of both T and B lymphocytes?

a) Antibody to CD3
b) Concanavalin A (ConA)
c) Phytohemagglutinin (PHA)
d) Pokeweed mitogen (PWM)
e) Certain strains of *Staphylococcus aureus*

50. Which of the following statements is TRUE of eukaryotic RNA polymerases?

a) They differ from prokaryotic RNA polymerases in that they also have an inherent ligase activity
b) They are similar to reverse transcriptase in that they utilize a DNA template
c) Three separate enzymes are used to synthesize each species of RNA (messenger, ribosomal, and transfer)
d) A single species of polymerase is used to synthesize rRNA, but several different species of polymerase are used to synthesize tRNA and mRNA
e) Transfer RNA and rRNA are synthesized by the same enzyme, but several different species of polymerase are used to make mRNA

51. Given the following statement: «.... a disease is uncommon in a population. It is incurable but seldom fatal ...» It is correct in this instance, for a given year that:

a) incidence is greater than prevalence
b) prevalence is greater than incidence
c) incidence and prevalence are equal
d) mortality rate is equal to infection rate
e) mortality rate is equal to prevalence

52. All of the following illnesses are more common among members of low socioeconomic status (SES) EXCEPT:

a) major depression
b) schizophrenia
c) obesity
d) high blood pressure
e) sexually-transmitted disease

53. While in the hospital following an appendectomy, a 29 year-old man frequently pouts and whines, and talks childishly to the medical staff. The ego defenses mechanism that he is using is:

a) rationalization
b) projection
c) repression
d) denial
e) regression

54. The aspect of the mind responsible for reality testing is:

a) the id
b) the ego
c) the superego
d) the preconscious
e) the unconscious

55. Which of the following reactions in the biosynthetic pathway for steroid hormones occurs in the endoplasmic reticulum?

a) Pregnenolone to progesterone
b) Corticosterone to aldosterone
c) 11-Deoxycortisol to cortisol
d) Cholesterol to pregnenolone
e) 17-α-OH progesterone to androstenedione

56. A dysfunction of nucleotide excision repair may cause a diversity of clinical conditions. An example of such condition or disease is:

a) hairy cell leukemia
b) HIV infection
c) alopecia
d) colorectal cancer
e) human papillomavirus infection (HPV)

57. The oxygen affinity in an oxygen transport protein, tends to increase in each of the following conditions, EXCEPT:

a) using myoglobin rather than hemoglobin
b) using a transport protein with a lower P_{50}
c) decreasing the partial pressure of carbon dioxide (pCO_2)
d) increasing the pH
e) increasing the concentration of 2,3 diphosphoglycerate (2,3-DPG)

58. The highest quantity of carbon dioxide in venous blood is present in the form of:

a) dissolved (gaseous)
b) bicarbonate (HCO_3-)
c) carbonic acid (H_2CO_3)
d) oxygen bound (O_2-CO_2)
e) carbaminohemoglobin (Hb-CO_2)

59. Which of the following statements regarding the mRNAs of both viruses and mammalian cells is INCORRECT?

a) Viral and cellular mRNAs are translated according to the same code
b) Viral and cellular mRNAs both have a 5' GTP cap
c) Viral and cellular mRNAs both have a 3' adenosine tail
d) Viral and cellular mRNAs are both transcribed using shifting reading frames
e) Viral and cellular mRNAs are both generated by splicing from a larger transcript of the genome

60. Which of the following vaccines uses a toxoid as the challenging antigen?

a) *Corynebacterium diphtheria* vaccine
b) *Bordetella pertussis* vaccine
c) *Salmonella typhi* vaccine
d) *Mycobacterium bovis* vaccine
e) *Vibrio cholera* vaccine

61. In which area of the brain might norepinephrine (NE) be found in high concentration?

a) Locus ceruleus
b) Raphe nucleus
c) Tuberinfundibular tract
d) Mucleus basalis
e) Nigrostriatal tract

USMLE step 1

BASIC MEDICAL SCIENCES

BOOK F TEST 6

Questions: 90 Time: 90 minutes

1. A 58-year-old smoker whitw male with chronic bronchitis and chronic obstructive pulmonary disease (COPD) is admitted to the hospital for multilobar pneumonia. In the culture of his sputum was isolated a gram negative rod which grew on heated-blood agar, in presence of factor X and factor V. The following antibiotics are effective in the treatment of this clinical condition, EXCEPT:

a) penicillin G
b) second generation cephalosporins
c) third generation cephalosporins
d) chloramphenicol
e) sulfamethoxazole/trimethoprim (bactrim)

2. Each of the following statements concerning the structure of carbohydrates is correct, EXCEPT:

a) maltose consists of two glucose molecules in an α(1,4) linkage
b) Sucrose consists of a glucose and a fructose molecule in an α(1,2) linkage
c) lactose consists of two galactose molecules in a ß(1,4) linkage
d) glycogen is a homopolysaccharide of glucose molecules linked by α(1,4) and α(1,6) bonds.
e) starch is found in plants and consists of amylopectin and amylose

3. Which of the following enzymes is deficient in the intestinal plasma membrane in the greatest percentage of the human population?

a) Trehalase
b) Oligo-1,6-glucosidase
c) α-glucosidase
d) ß-glucosidase
e) ß-galactosidase

4. A protodiastolic gallop rhythm (S_3/S_4 gallop) is most likely the result of:

a) a loss of ventricular compliance
b) a prolapsed mitral valve
c) an aortic valvular stenosis
d) a ruptured papillary muscle
e) a healthy 25 year-old male during moderate exercise

5. During blood pressure measurement on an apparently healthy 28-year-old woman, a third year student deflates the cuff to a reading of 96 mmHg before a sharp «thud» is heard; the radial pulse becomes palpable at this pressure. Which of the following is the best interpretation of these findings?

a) The systolic pressure is 96 mmHg
b) The diastolic pressure is 96 mmHg
c) The auscultatory gap occurs at 96 mmHg
d) The sphingomanometer is defective
e) A heart murmur is present

Items 6-7

Item 6

A patient with Parkinson's disease was being successfully treated with L-dopa alone. After he began taking a daily multiple vitamin preparation, his symptoms of Parkinson's disease began to worsen. The best explanation is:

a) vitamin A is an inhibitor of the dopamine neuronal transporter
b) vitamin B_1 can antagonize dopamine receptors
c) vitamin B_1 competes for plasma binding and accelerates the degradation of L-dopa
d) vitamin B_6 is a co-factor for the decarboxylation of L-dopa
e) vitamin D accumulates in the substantia nigra

Item 7

The most appropriate treatment for the above patient would be:

a) carbidopa plus L-dopa
b) selegiline plus L-dopa
c) bromocriptine plus L-dopa
d) trihexylphenidine plus L-dopa
e) increase the dosage of L-dopa

8. Hexokinase I:

a) is found primarily in the liver
b) catalyzes the hydrolysis of glucose into two 3-carbon fragments
c) has a higher specificity for glucose than does glucokinase
d) has a higher KM for glucose than does glucokinase
e) is essentially saturated at normal blood glucose levels

9. Which of the following enzymes used in glycolysis requires the investment of ATP?

a) Phosphoglucoisomerase (PGI)
b) Phosphofructokinase (PFK)
c) Pyruvate kinase (PK)
d) Phosphoglycerate kinase (PGK)
e) Aldolase

10. Which of the following events is most likely to be involved in triggering ovulation?

a) The presence of a corpus luteum
b) Continuous release of high levels of gonadotropin releasing hormone (GnRH)
c) Pulsatile release of high levels of GnRH
d) Continuous release of high levels of progesterone
e) Pulsatile release of high levels of FSH

11. Type I (red) muscle fibers:

a) are innervated by large nerves
b) have a greater sarcoplasmic reticulum pumping capacity than type II fibers
c) have a glycolytic capacity higher than oxidative capacity
d) have a fast myosin isozyme
e) produce slow and prolonged contractions

Items 12-14

Match the following drugs used to treat acid peptic disorders with the descriptions below.

a) Propantheline
b) Cimetidine
c) Misoprostol
d) Omeprazole
e) None of the above

12. It is a muscarinic receptor antagonist which promotes mucosal healing by blocking the vagus nerve.

13. It is an analog of prostaglandin E_1, with antisecretory and cytoprotective properties.

14. It inhibits the gastric H^+/K^+-ATPase, a membrane-bound proton pump. It is effective in the management of gastric acid hypersecretion.

15. The measles virus has been found to increase IL-4 production and decrease IL-2 and gamma IFN production. Which of the following is the most likely result of these effects?

a) A substantial decline in cell-mediated immunity (CMI)
b) A substantial decline in humoral immunity
c) A substantial decline in both CMI and humeral immunity
d) A hyperreactive CMI response
e) An increased in the production of antigen-presenting cells (APC)

16. Which of the following events is LEAST likely to occur following binding of ligand to the fibroblast growth factor receptor (FGFR)?

a) Endocytosis
b) Localization of FGF to the nucleus
c) Autophosphorylation of tyrosine residues on the receptor
d) Phosphorylation of intracellular proteins
e) Receptor dimerization

17. Which of the following nucleotide phosphates is most directly involved in glycoside synthesis?

a) UDP
b) CTP
c) TDP
d) AMP
e) GTP

18. Compared to adults, which of the following patterns is correct regarding healthy infants?

	Heart rate	**Blood pressure**
a)	No change	Increased
b)	Increased	Decreased
c)	Increased	Increased
d)	Decreased	No change
e)	No change	Decreased

19. Biotransformation of drugs may produce metabolites which are active, inactive, or toxic as compared to the parent compound. Of the drugs below, which is converted to a toxic rather than an active metabolite?

a) Heroin
b) Diazepam
c) Codeine
d) Halothane
e) Prednisone

Items 20-21

Item 20

A man with severe duodenal ulcers and gastric acid hypersecretion is diagnosed with Zollinger Ellison syndrome. This results from a tumor derived of the:

a) gastric chief cells
b) gastric parietal cells
c) intestinal Paneth cells
d) pancreatic islet cells
e) hepatocytes

Item 21

The features of this tumor are the following, EXCEPT:

a) is a G-cells tumor
b) is second in frequency after insulinomas
c) is common between the ages of 30 and 50 years
d) may rise from duodenal tissue
e) can produce mild diabetes and erythematous necrotizing, and migratory rash

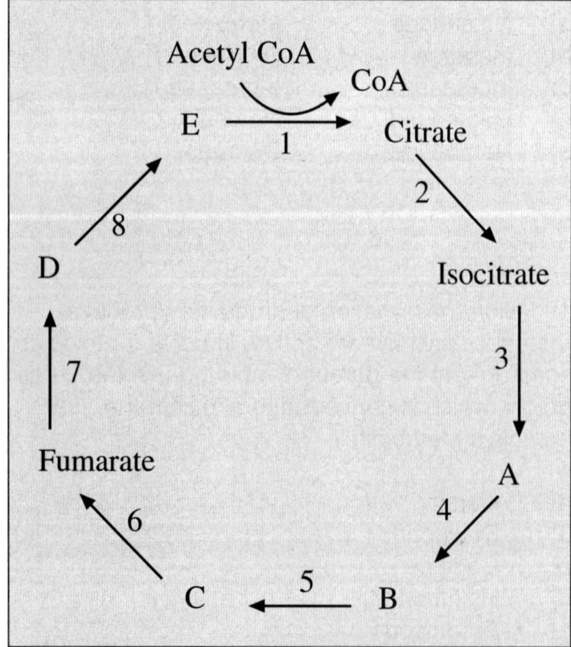

Figure 42 (Question 6.25)

Items 22-23

Select the best answer from the following list.

a) Proproxyphene
b) Phenobarbital
c) Dextroamphetamine
d) Diazepam
e) Chloropromazine

22. It is a neuroleptic drug useful in the treatment of psychotic symptoms.

23. It is a derivative of methadone, used as an analgesic to relieve mild to moderate pain.

24. Which of the following enzymes are utilized in gluconeogenesis but NOT in glycolysis?

a) Pyruvate transaminase and triose-phosphate isomerase
b) Pyruvate kinase and phophoenolpyruvate carboxykinase
c) Fructose bisphosphatase and phosphoenolpyruvate carboxykinase
d) Phosphofructokinase and pyruvate carboxylase
e) Malate dehydrogenase and aldolase

Items 25-28

Answer the following questions concerning the citric acid cycle, depicted in the figure 42.

25. High-energy intermediate which drives the formation of GTP.

26. The only five-carbon intermediate in the cycle.

27. According the diagram of the figure 42, the enzyme dehydrogenase which produces $FADH_2$ is:

a) 3
b) 4
c) 5
d) 6
e) 7

28. According the figure 42, which is the enzyme catalyzing the most endergonic reaction of the cycle, producing a forward reaction favored by low product concentration.

a) 1
b) 2
c) 5
d) 7
e) 8

Items 29-30

The columns in the table below show the sequence of reactions in the metabolism of hemoglobin. Use the trends in changes of pigment levels to identify the specific type of jaundice.

	Bilirubin (BR)	BR-albumin	BR-diglucuronide	Urobilin
a)	normal	normal	increased	decreased
b)	normal	decreased	increased	decreased
c)	increased	increased	increased	increased
d)	increased	decreased	normal	increased
e)	normal	increased	decreased	decreased

29. Obstructive jaundice.

30. Hemolytic jaundice.

31. A 49 year old white female is being treated with chemotherapy for breast cancer. She has a history of frequent and refractory nauseas and vomiting and you decided to place her on dronabinol (marinol. All of the following can be expected during the therapeutic use of this medicine, EXCEPT:

a) decreases the effects of sympathomimetics and tricyclic drugs
b) uptake and distribution more prolonged with oral than intravenous administration
c) hepatic biotransformation yields multiple hydroxylated metabolites, which may be either active or inactive
d) a decrease in nausea and vomiting associated with cancer chemotherapy
e) the drug and its lipid-soluble metabolites may be sequestered in body fat

Items 32-34

Match the following diseases with their biochemical basis.

a) Maple syrup urine disease
b) Homocystinuria
c) Cystic fibrosis (CF)
d) Phenylketonuria (PKU)
e) Lesch-Nyhan syndrome

32. A defective transmembrane conductance regulator.

33. Decreased capacity to metabolize valine.

34. Decreased reutilization of a precursor for inosine monophosphate (IMP).

35. To complete gluconeogenesis, shuttle mechanisms exist for the transport of intermediates. Which of the following best describes such a shuttle system?

a) Oxaloacetate is converted to aspartate which is transported across the outer mitochondrial membrane
b) Pyruvate is converted to lactate which is transported across the plasma membrane
c) Malate is converted to alpha-ketoglutarate which is transported across the inner mitochondrial membrane
d) Phosphoenolpyruvate is converted to malate which is transported across the inner mitochondrial membrane
e) Glutamate is converted to oxaloacetate which is transported across the outer mitochondrial membrane

36. It is noticed that, when interested or afraid, a cat's pupils become larger. Which system is most likely responsible for this observation?

a) Sympathetic system
b) Parasympathetic system
c) Somatic nervous system
d) Dopaminegeric system
e) Increased serotonin conductance

37. Figure 43 shows the results of a polyacrylamide gel electrophoresis experiment. Two samples of a radiolabelled plasmid X were loaded into the gel. Lane A contains a sample of plasmid X. Lane B contains a sample of plasmid X which had undergone an experimental manipulation prior to loading. Which of the following experimental manipulations of plasmid X most plausibly explains the differences observed between lanes A and B?

a) Plasmid X was fragmented with a restriction endonuclease
b) Plasmid X was diluted in deionized water.
c) Plasmid X was treated with a topoisomerase to induce supercoiling.
d) Plasmid X was ligated with another piece of DNA
e) Plasmid X underwent replication.

38. The DNA in the gel electrophoresis of a DNA sample:

a) is positively charged and hence moves toward the anode
b) is positively charged and hence moves toward the cathode
c) is negatively charged and hence moves toward the anode
d) is negatively charged and hence moves toward the cathode
e) the movement is unrelated to charge

39. Each of the following statements regarding the structural components of lipids is correct, EXCEPT:

a) a sphingosine is a condensation of an amino acid and a fatty acid
b) a ceramide is a sphingosine with an amide linkage to a fatty acid
c) sphingomyelin consists of a phosphocholine molecule combined with a ceramide molecule
d) a ganglioside consists of a fatty acid conjugated to guanosine triphosphate
e) in adipocytes, fatty acids are stored conjugated into glycerol

40. Which of the following lipids is present in the greatest amount in the human erythrocyte membrane?

a) Phosphatidylcholine
b) Phosphatidylinositol
c) Cholesterol
d) Sphingomyelin
e) Glycolipid

Figure 43 (Question 6.37)

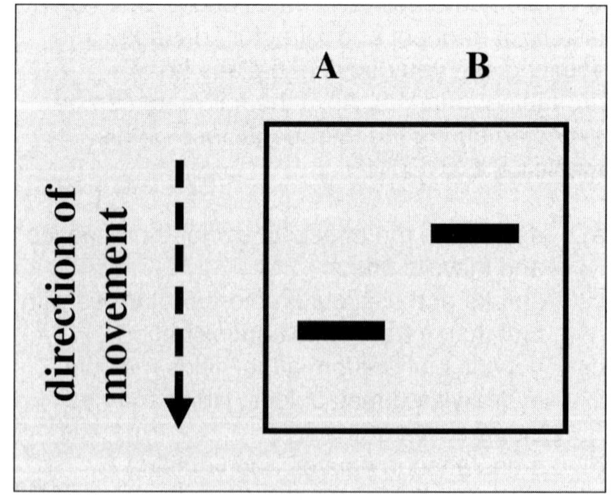

Items 41-42

Answer the following questions regarding the enzyme and their serum levels used clinically to evaluate myocardial infarction (MI).

a) Asparate transaminase (AST)
b) Alanine transaminase (ALT)
c) Troponin T
d) Creatine kinase (CK)
e) Lactic dehydrogenase (LDH)

41. This enzyme may remain elevated up to two weeks following an MI.

42. Exists as an isozyme; if levels remain elevated more than four days after an MI, an extension (second MI) is likely.

Items 43-45

a) Hydralazine
b) Procainamide
c) Nitroglycerin
d) Verapamil
e) None of the above

43. It is useful in treating arrhythmias such as ventricular tachycardia.

44. The antihypertensive effect derives from selectivity for adrenergic receptors.

45. Vasodilator drug used in congestive heart failure with lupus erythematosus-like side effects.

46. An overdose of which of the following drugs might be treated with monoclonal antibodies?

a) Amitriptyline
b) Atropine
c) Digoxin
d) Lithium
e) Secobarbitol

47. Pyruvate may be directly converted in a single step to each of the following compounds, EXCEPT:

a) lactate
b) acetaldehyde
c) glutamate
d) oxaloacetate
e) acetyl CoA

Items 48-49

Select the best answer from the list below.

a) DNA footprinting
b) Mobility shift DNA binding assay
c) Oligo-nucleotide mutagenesis
d) Linker scanning mutagenesis
e) Enzyme-linked immunosorbant assay (ELISA)

48. It alters a DNA sequence in a defined way.

49. It can be used to locate the specific binding site of a protein on DNA.

50. A large tumor of the uncinate process of the pancreas is most likely to obstruct which of the following veins?

a) Splenic vein
b) Middle colic vein
c) Inferior epigastric vein
d) Renal vein
e) Gastroepiploic vein

51. Heart bypass surgery is performed to circumvent a nearly occluded marginal branch of the right coronary artery. Which of the following veins is in closest proximity to the marginal artery?

a) Great cardiac vein
b) Middle cardiac vein
c) Small cardiac vein
d) Anterior cardiac vein
e) Thesbian vein

52. Which of the following veins is a landmark for distinguishing direct versus indirect inguinal hernias?

a) Inferior epigastric
b) Internal iliac
c) External iliac
d) Inferior vesicular
e) Testicular

53. General anesthetics:

a) act by binding to specific receptors.
b) with low blood : gas solubility tend to equilibrate rapidly
c) the equilibration of those with high blood : gas solubility tends to be limited by cardiac output rather than respiratory rate
d) agents such as halothane and enflurane are typically injected intravenously rather than inhaled
e) none of the above

54. Each of the following are positive inotropic agents EXCEPT:

a) amrinone
b) dipyridimole
c) dobutamine
d) caffeine
e) bretylium

Items 55-56

a) Clomiphene
b) Mestranol
c) Tamoxifen
d) Ethinyl estradiol
e) Norethindrone

55. It is useful in treating some forms of breast cancer.

56. A 29-year-old woman delivers triplets after having been on a regimen of this drug.

57. The Cori cycle is most likely to:

a) decrease glucose levels in skeletal muscle
b) convert pyruvate to triacylglycerol
c) utilize lipoprotein lipase
d) transport lactate from muscle to liver
e) synthesize unsaturated fatty acid through a glyoxylate intermediate

58. An experiment demonstrates that the molecular weight of glycogen increases when a specific, soluble enzyme inhibitor is added to cultured hepatocytes. The inhibitor most likely decreases the activity of:

a) glycogen synthetase b
b) glycogen synthase kinase-3
c) protein phosphatase I
d) glycogen phosphorylase b
e) glycogen phosphorylase kinase

59. A 4-year-old girl presents with hepatomegaly and chronic hypoglycemia. The liver biopsy reveals abnormally long, unbranched chains of glycogen. The glycogen storage disease which afflicts this patient is most likely:

a) type I (von Gierke's)
b) type II (Pompe's)
c) type III (Cori's).
d) type IV (Anderson's)
e) type V (McArdle-Schmidt-Pearson's)

60. Which of the following fatty acids has the highest ratio of number of double bonds to number of carbon atoms?

a) Linoleic
b) Myristate
c) Oleate
d) Palmitate
e) Stearate

61. Which of the following techniques would be most appropriate for separating a mixture of proteins on the basis of molecular weight?

a) Gel filtration chromatography
b) Ion-exchange chromatography
c) Affinity chromatography
d) Metal-chelate chromatography
e) High pressure chromatofocusing

62. Using immunohistochemistry, you have determined that protein X is located intracellularly in a culture of embryonic fibroblasts. Which of the following techniques would be the best way to determine whether protein X is synthesized as well as stored in this cell line?

a) Fractional ultracentrifugation
b) Western blotting
c) In situ hybridization
d) Electron microscopy
e) Fluorescent monoclonal antibodies

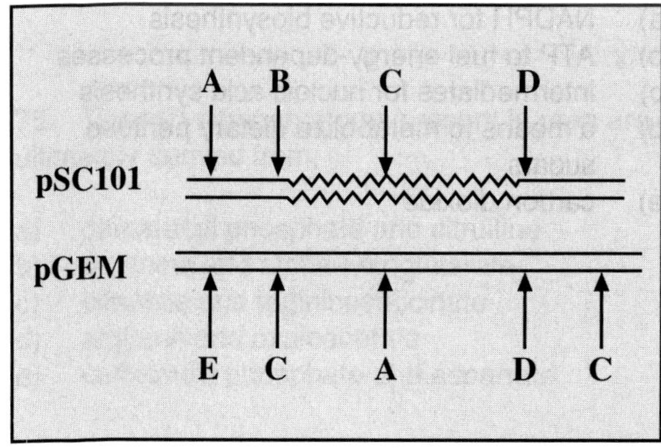

Figure 44 (Question 6.63)

Items 63-64

The figure 44 depicts a 1.2 kB gene of interest (jagged line) in a pSC101 plasmid vector (5.5 kB total) and a second plasmid, pGEM (7.0 kB). Both are circular plasmids (depicted linearly for clarity.) The arrows show the location of restriction sites on each plasmid (each different letter represents a different restriction enzyme). Each enzyme cleave to yield cohesive ends.

63. It is decided to subclone this gene into an expression plasmid, pGEM. Which combination of restriction enzymes would afford the simplest means to transfer the gene from pSC101 into pGEM such that an active protein may subsequently be expressed?

a) Enzymes A and D
b) Enzymes B and D
c) Enzymes E, B and D
d) Enzymes A, B, and C
e) Enzymes A, B, C, and D

64. The plasmids are treated with the proper enzymes and the gene of interest is ligated into pGEM. An agarose gel electrophoresis is run on the reaction mixture, and five bands are seen and their lengths are determined. The band of which of the following sizes is mostly likely to contain the recombinant plasmid (pGEM plus the gene of interest)?

a) 1.2 kB
b) 3.7 kB
c) 7.6 kB
d) 9.1 kB
e) 12.5kB

Item 78

It is decided to analyze the rat embryonic fibroblasts to determine the levels of messenger RNA encoding a specific receptor for ligand C before and after treatment with hormone P. Which of the following techniques will be most useful in this experiment?

a) Northern blotting
b) Southern blotting
c) Western blotting
d) High pressure liquid chromatography (HPLC)
e) Isoelectric focusing

79. A patient with carpal tunnel syndrome is most likely to experience which of the following symptoms?

a) Flexion of the wrist and weakness of the finger muscles
b) Paresthesia of the index, middle and fourth fingers
c) Paresthesia of the thumb, index, middle, and medial side of the fourth fingers and thenar weakness
d) Flexion of the fourth and fifth fingers into a claw-like posture and weakness and paresthesia over the hypothenar region
e) Intermittent pain and paralysis of the hand

80. A line perpendicular to the long axis of the body passed through the sternal angle (of Louis) will intersect which of the following vertebrae?

a) C7
b) T1
c) T2
d) T3
e) T4

81. A child is born with syndactyly or fused fingers. Failure of which of the following developmental processes is most likely responsible?

a) Migration
b) Differentiation
c) Apoptosis
d) Mitosis
e) Gastrulation

82. How much energy is produced from metabolizing 5 grams of protein, 8 grams of carbohydrate, and 6 grams of fat?

a) 87 kcal
b) 96 kcal
c) 106 kcal
d) 141 kcal
e) 190 kcal

83. Which of the following statements regarding the enzymes that regulate triglyceride storage and mobilization is CORRECT?

a) Hormone-sensitive lipase and acyl CoA synthetase are located at the adipocyte plasma membrane
b) Lipoprotein lipase releases free fatty acids and glycerol from triglycerides
c) Hormone-sensitive lipase is activated by insulin and inhibited by epinephrine
d) Insulin acts to increase blood levels of fatty acids
e) Transport of dietary fat to adipocytes is regulated more tightly than is mobilization of fat from storage depots

84. The figure 45 depicts the plasma levels in arbitrary units of three different substances during the course of an experimental ten-day fasting period. According this graph, which of the following statements is most likely to be TRUE?

a) «A» represents ketone bodies and «B» represents glucose
b) «A» represents lactate and «C» represents glucose
c) «B» represents fatty acids and «C» represents ketone bodies
d) «A» represents insulin and «B» represents glucagon
e) «A» represents glucose-6-phosphate and «B» represents glycogen

85. What are the products of ß-oxidation of an unsaturated 17-carbon fatty acid?

a) Eight pyruvate molecules and one acetaldehyde molecule
b) Four oxaloacetate molecules and one methyl CoA molecule
c) Four malate molecules and one carbon dioxide
d) Seven acetyl-CoA molecules and one propionyl CoA molecule
e) Seven pyruvate molecules and one dihydroxyacetone phosphate molecule

Figure 45 (Question 6.84)

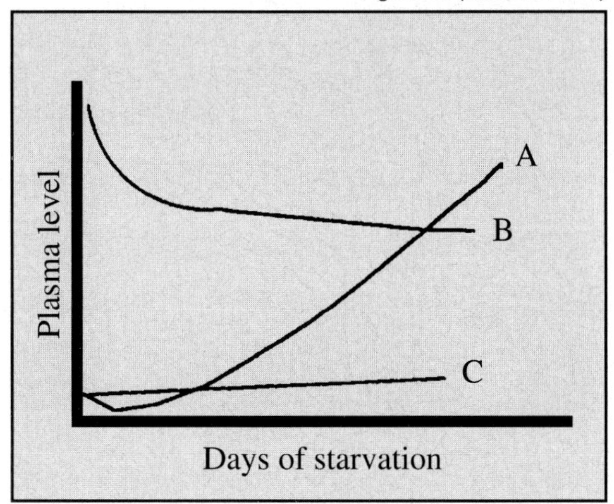

86. Refsum's disease is a severe congenital neurological disorder caused by a defect in lipid metabolism. Patients with this condition accumulate large amounts of phytanic acid. Which of the following dietary measures should be taken to minimize the symptoms of this disease?

a) Avoid long-chain (C12-C18) fatty acids
b) Avoid medium-chain (C6-C12) fatty acids
c) Avoid cholesterol and low-density lipoprotein
d) Avoid foods containing ketogenic amino acids
e) Avoid foods containing chlorophyll.

87. Which of the following tendons passes behind the lateral malleolus?

a) Flexor digitorum longus
b) Tibialis posterior
c) Flexor hallucis longus
d) Peroneus brevis
e) Peroneus tertius

88. Which of the following statement regarding the vascularization around the spinal cord is CORRECT?

a) The anterior and posterior spinal arteries travel in the vertebral foramen
b) The anterior spinal artery is unpaired and supplies the anterior 2/3 of the spinal cord
c) The posterior spinal artery is unpaired and supplies the posterior 1/3 of the spinal cord
d) The posterior spinal artery travels through the transverse foraminae of the first six cervical vertebrae
e) The posterior spinal arteries are paired and supply the posterior 2/3 of the spinal cord

89. During surgery in the neck, the external carotid artery is tied off just proximal to the bifurcation of the lingual artery. As a result, blood flow will be decreased through all of the following arteries, EXCEPT the:

a) facial artery
b) posterior auricular artery
c) occipital artery
d) maxillary artery
e) ascending pharyngeal artery

90. Each of the following correctly pairs an inherited disease of sphingolipid catabolism with the defective enzyme, EXCEPT:

	Disease	**Enzyme**
a)	Tay-Sachs Disease	ß-N-acetylhexosaminidase A
b)	Niemann-Pick Disease	sphingomyelinase
c)	Metachromatic leukodystrophy	arylsulfatase A
d)	GM1 gangliosidosis	ß-galactosidase
e)	Gaucher's disease	ß-glucuronidase

USMLE step 1

BASIC MEDICAL SCIENCES

BOOK F TEST 1

ANSWERS

1.E

G-C pairs contain three hydrogen bonds and thus are held together more strongly than A-T pairs, which contain two hydrogen bonds. Incubation at high temperature, extremes of pH, or with certain enzymes favors strand separation (denaturation).

2.B

The first heart sound results from the closure of the atrioventricular valves. The second heart sound results from the closure of the aortic and pulmonic valves.

3.B; 4.C; 5.D; 6.C

Digitoxin and digoxin are cardiac glycosides which are useful in clinical settings such as congestive heart failure. Both enhance myocardial excitation-contraction coupling to increase cardiac excitability, speed conduction velocity. **Digitoxin** is highly absorbed and bound (97%), and is metabolized by the liver (where ten percent of the active drug is converted to digoxin). It has a long half-life of 7 days. In contrast, Digoxin is less well absorbed and less bound to plasma proteins (25%), giving it a shorter half-life (36 h). Digoxin is excreted unchanged by the kidneys. **Captopril** inhibits the action of the angiotensin converting enzyme, therefore diminishes the inactivation of bradykinin. It causes vasodilation and lowers peripheral vascular resistance, causing a decrease in blood pressure. It also decreases the circulating levels of aldosterone, decreases retention of sodium and fluid, and increases the retention of potassium. The combined above effects improve the symptoms of congestive heart failure. **Propranolol** is a beta-adrenergic blocker drug. It diminishes cardiac output, having both negative inotropic and chronotropic effects. It is used in angina pectoris because it reduces the oxygen requirement of the heart muscle, therefore it reduces the chest pain. It has a protective effect on the myocardium, reduces infarct size and quickens recovery after myocardial necrosis.

7.E

The foramen rotundum transmits the maxillary nerve. The foramen spinosum transmits middle meningeal artery and vein. The foramen ovale transmits the mandibular nerve and accessory meningeal artery. The internal carotid artery passes over the foramen lacerum (which is covered by cartilege). The superior orbital fissure transmits the oculomotor, trochlear, and abducens nerves and the ophthalmic nerve and vein.

8.E

The stage of concrete operations (which follows the preoperational stage and precedes formal operations) is characterized by logical thought.

9.C

The Sanger DNA sequencing method is based upon random insertion of 2',3'-ddNTPs in a growing DNA chain specified by the template of interest. The ddNTPs have a normal 5'-phosphate, and are thus incorporated into the strand. However, because they lack a 3' hydroxyl group, they prevent the incorporation of further bases. By running four separate reactions (one for each nucleotide - A, G, C, and T) and adjusting the reaction conditions, a series of labeled strands of different lengths is generated. When subjected to electrophoresis, the DNA sequence may be deduced.

10.C

A split S_2 is a normal finding on auscultation. It represents the earlier closure of the aortic valve versus the pulmonic valve due to higher pressure and earlier depolarization in the left side of the heart. It is best heard at the peak of inspiration.

11.D

The antigen binding site is found at the ends of the «arms» of the immunoglobulin molecule. It is formed by the variable regions of both the light and heavy chains.

12.C

Creutzfield-Jakob disease is caused by a slow virus which produces no inflammatory response. It is transmitted from human-to-human through infected brain tissue during corneal transplantation, contaminated neurosurgical instruments, or prescription of growth hormone from cadaver pituitary. Dementia and a variety of motor and sensory signs may occur. It is incurable and fatal usually within a year of the onset of symptoms.

13.B

An apical lung (Pancoast's) tumor may cause shortness of breath and bloody sputum. Moreover, sympathetic fibers from the superior cervical ganglion, which may descend as low as the thoracic vertebrae, may be compressed. The result is Horner's syndrome, which consists of ptosis (drooping eyelid), miosis (pupillary constriction due to unopposed parasympathetic action), and anhydrosis (lack of sweat production).

14.E

Stress decreases every measurable parameter of immune responsivity. Moreover, corticosteroids, which also depress the immune system, are produced in higher amounts during stress. Stimulation of the anterior hypothalamus enhances immune responsivity, while stimulation of the posterior hypothalamus inhibits immune activity.

15.E

The trochlear nerve (CN IV) controls the contralateral superior oblique muscle, hence the left superior oblique is controlled by the right trochlear nerve. Injury of this nerve results in extortion (outward rotation), diplopia, and weakness in downward and lateral gaze. A patient with a trochlear nerve palsy can obtain binocular vision by tilting his/her head to the unaffected side.

16.D

Natural (innate) immunity is nonspecific and includes physical barriers (skin and mucus membranes), cells, proteins, and processes such as inflammation and phagocytosis.

17.B

The muscles of facial expression are innervated by CN VII, the nucleus of which is located in the caudal (tegemental) part of the pons. CN IX-XII arise from the medulla, IV-VII arise from the pons, and III and IV arise from the midbrain. CN I and II arise from forebrain nuclei. Fibers from CN II-VI travel through the cavernous sinus.

18.C

Tolerance, a lack of response to a specific antigen is favored by a simple antigenic structure, by very large or very small doses of antigen, and by using aggregated antigens or adjuvants. Neonatal animals, and animals on immunosuppressive drugs such as CsA (which suppresses IL-2 production) are also more likely to become tolerant.

19.C

Patients with hippocampal lesions are often unable to remember events which happened thirty minutes ago, but may have intact long-term memories.

20.D

The onset of anorexia nervosa is nearly always between the ages of 10 and 30, and it is 10-20 times more common in females. It involves the false perception that one is obese. Amenorrhea or absence of at least three consecutive menstrual cycles, is in the diagnostic criteria. Despite the name, appetite is normal until late in the disorder. It is fatal in 9% of the cases.

21.A

Taq polymerase is derived from *Thermicus aquaticus*, a bacteria which lives in hot springs. It has a temperature optimum of 72°C; enzymes from most other bacteria work best at temperatures under 40°C. The higher temperatures increase the binding specificity of the primers. Moreover, the enzyme is not denatured during the repeated cycles of heating (to denature) and cooling (to reanneal) the strands of DNA.

22.C

Systemic vascular resistance is decreased at all stages of pregnancy as compared to pre-pregnancy levels, and drops sharply at delivery. Heart rate, stroke volume, and blood volume increase during the first trimester and peak in the second trimester before decreasing. Left ventricular end diastolic pressure remains largely unchanged.

23.B

Trazodone is an antidepressant thought to act by selectively inhibiting serotonin uptake by brain synaptosomes. It is associated with orthostatic hypotension and priapism.

24.B

The unpaired anterior spinal artery travels in the anterior spinal sulcus and supplies the anterior 2/3 of the spinal cord. The paired posterior spinal arteries travel near the spinal nerve roots and supply the posterior 1/3 of the spinal cord. The spinal cord travels in the vertebral foramen, and the vertebral arteries travel in the transverse foraminae.

25.A

Bleuler also described accessory symptoms of schizophrenia, including hallucinations, impaired language, judgment, and coordination, and involuntary movements.

26.D

The stem-loop structure in the figure forms because of internally complimentary base pairing. Beginning from the ends of the molecule and reading inward, it is clear that each G is paired with a C and each A with a U.

27.E

Methadone is an opioid similar to morphine but with a longer half life (15 h). It is effective orally and has an abuse potential similar to morphine. It is used to suppress the withdrawal symptoms of heroin dependent individuals.

28.A

Biotransformation of drugs occurs in two phases. **Phase 1** involves chemical modification (oxidation, hydroxylation, etc.) to a more polar intermediate. **Phase 2** involves conjugation with water-soluble compounds. Acetaminophen (like chloramphenicol and others) is conjugated to glucuronic acid. Compounds B-E are conjugated to acetyl-CoA; there are at least two isozymes of the enzyme catalyzing this reaction (N-acetyl transferase), giving rise to «slow» and «fast» acetylators.

29.D

Condoms and diaphragms act as barriers to human papilloma virus (HPV), which may explain the decreased incidence of cervical neoplasia. Users of oral contraceptives seem to have higher rates of cervical cancer, hepatic adenoma, and gallstones, but lower rates of ovarian and endometrial cancer. There seems to be no significant risk of sterility following the use of transdermal patches. Each method has a failure rate: oral contraceptives (0.27%/year), diaphragm (1.9%), condoms (3.6%), spermicidal foam (11.9%), and cervical cap (8-17%).

30.C

Normal bacterial flora can cause disease but also serve important protective and nutritive functions. The urinary bladder is normally sterile, though urine may become contaminated with *S. epidermidis* as it passes through the distal urethra.

31.D

Cloninger described three heritable dimensions of personality. Novelty-seeking was correlated with the dopaminergic system, harm avoidance with serotonin, and reward dependence with norepinephrine. This system is probably an oversimplification.

32.C

The kappa light, lambda light, and heavy chain genes are located on chromosomes 2, 22, and 14 respectively. Each type of chain obtains genes from a separate pool. Light chains are formed by splicing together one V gene (variable, 100-200 genes in the pool), one J gene (junction, 6 genes) and one C gene (constant, 1 gene for either kappa or lambda). Heavy chains also incorporate a D gene (diversity, 6 genes) between V and J; there are 9 C genes (one for each antibody class).

33.B, 34.A

An experiment bridging gray and white matter with intercostal nerve bridges was recently performed on rats with spinal cord transections. The connections were stabilized with FGF-fibrin. The rats showed a partial restoration of hind limb function.

35.B

Idiotypes are the antigenic determinants in the hypervariable region. Isotypes are determined by the constant regions of heavy and light chain (e.g., IgG vs. IgM, kappa vs. lambda light chain). Allotypes vary between individuals and consist of additional antigenic features of immunoglobulins. A haplotype is the set of HLA (human leukocyte antigens) expressed by an individual.

36.D; 37.B; 38.C

The *tat* gene encodes a protein which acts as a transcriptional activator; *vpr* also encodes a transcriptional activator. The polymerase gene (*pol*) encodes viral enzymes, including reverse transcriptase and integrase. *Rev* binds to a rev response element (RRE), which removes a block in the transport of unspliced RNAs out of the nucleus. The *nef* gene seems to function in maintaining a high level of infectivity; the *vif* gene also increases infectivity of viral particles. The *vpu* gene participates in viral assembly and budding.

39.C

Acquired immunity may be **active** when induced after contact with foreign antigens or **passive** when antibodies preformed in another host. Passive immunity has a rapid onset but induces no memory and carries the risk of an allergic response.

40.B

A «pulled groin» is an injury caused by excessive tension on the adductor muscles (magnus, longus, and brevis) at their tendinous origins around the obturator foramen.

41.C

Erection/vaginal lubrication occur during the excitement phase. During the plateau, there is hyperventilation and increased blood pressure. Orgasm is an involuntary series of sphincter contractions. During resolution, parameters return to normal.

42.C

The risk of mental illness increases with age, and is highest among the elderly. Sociopathy and schizophrenia are more common among men, and bipolar and anxiety disorders are more common among women.

43.A

Bipolar disorder is characterized by severe mood swings between depression and elation and by remission and recurrence. Episodes of depression and manic features (extreme fatigue with racing thoughts, hypersomnia) may present simultaneously. Emotional blunting with formal thought disturbances, disturbances of the subjective experience of self, disturbances of volition and behavior, ambivalence, and autism are typical features of schizophrenia.

44.D; 45.B

Organic phosphates and chloride are anions (negatively charged) while calcium, potassium, and sodium are cations (positively charged). Sodium and chloride are present in the highest molar concentrations in the extracellular fluid, while potassium and phosphates are the predominant intracellular ions.

46.B

There are eight interossei muscles in the hand, four dorsal and four palmar. Each is supplied by the deep branch of the ulnar nerve. The dorsal interossei abduct the fingers away from the third finger, and the palmar interossei adduct the fingers toward the third finger. In addition, both groups flex the metacarpophalangeal joints and extend the interphalangeal joints.

47.A

Reliability refers to the consistency of measurements, while validity refers to how accurately the intended parameter is measured. Sensitivity is the true positive rate, while specificity is the true negative rate.

48.B

In PCR, double-stranded DNA with a sequence to be amplified is denatured by heating, then cooled so that the primers annealed to binding regions which flank the target sequence. *Taq* polymerase is added, and the strands are duplicated. Following successive cycles of heating and cooling, the sequence between the primers is progressively amplified.

49.D

An Apgar score below seven suggests a high-risk neonatal situation. The score is determined as follows:

Sign	0	1	2
Heart rate	Absent	Below 100	Above 100
Respiratory effort	Absent	Slow, irregular	Good, crying
Color	Blue, pale	Body pink, extremities blue	Completely pink
Muscle tone	Flaccid	Some flexion	Active motion
Reflex irritability	Absent	Cry	Vigorous cry

50.C

Antibodies to polysaccharide capsules are used in vaccines for *S. pneumoniae, N. meningitides*, and *H. influenzae*. The capsule is external to the cell wall and prevents phagocytosis; it is the primary determinant of the serotype.

51.D

Decerebrate posturing is seen in a comatose patient with a brain injury between the vestibular nuclei in the floor of the fourth ventricle (involved in extension) and the red nuclei of the rostral midbrain tegmentum (involved in flexion, especially of the upper limbs). Flexion input is lost, hence both limbs are extended. In contrast, decorticate posturing involves damage above the red nuclei and is characterized by extension of the lower limbs and flexion of the upper limbs.

52.C; 53.A; 54.B

CT scanning remains the most widely available imaging modality. It provides better images in the transverse than the coronal or sagittal planes but has lower contrast resolution than MRI, and may produce imaging artifacts near dense bone. MRI operates by manipulating the electromagnetic forces in tissues. PET scans and single photon emission computed tomography (SPECT) scans are functional imaging techniques which can be used to analyze cerebral blood flow and metabolism.

55.D

The ABO blood groups are alloantigens on the surface of RBCs and other cells; they encode sugar transferases. A and B are codominant to O. The Rh(D) gene is another RBC marker, Rh(D)+ is dominant to Rh(D)-. In this case, the child could be the natural offspring of Ms. Y and Mr. X if Ms. Y's genotype is B/O, Rh(D)-/Rh(D)-, and the Mr. X's genotype is A/O, Rh(D)+/Rh(D)+ or -. The child's genotype is therefore O/O, Rh(D)+/Rh(D)-.

56.A; 57.D; 58.B; 59.A; 60.C

Heparin and warfarin are both used in anticoagulant therapy. **Heparin** is a naturally-occurring glycosaminoglycan which interacts with antithrombin III to inhibit thrombosis by inactivating factor X and inhibiting thrombin formation. Heparin is effective both in vivo and in vitro, and has not been found to cross the placenta, presumably due to its large size. It is typically administered intravenously or subcutaneously. **Warfarin** (coumarin) exerts its anticoagulant effects by inhibiting the gamma-carboxylation of the vitamin K-dependent clotting factors, factors II, VII, IX, and X. It works only in vivo, and is contraindicated in pregnancy. It is administered orally and is highly bound. **Aspirin** blocks thromboxane A_2 synthesis from arachidonic acid in platelets by irreversibly acetylating and thus inhibiting cyclo-oxygenase with suppression of the platelet aggregation for the life of the platelet. It is useful in the prophylactic treatment of transient cerebral ischemia, to reduce the incidence of recurrent myocardial infarction and to decrease mortality in postmyocardial infarction patients. **Ticlopidine** is an antiplatelet drug used in the prophylaxis of thrombotic stroke in selected patients intolerant to aspirin. It potentiates the activity of aspirin, anticoagulants, antipyrine, and theophylline. **Warfarin** is attenuated when it is used concomittant with barbiturates, glutethimine, griseofulvin and rifampin. Its effects can be potentiated with the concomitant use of cimetidine, cotrimoxazole, chloramphenicol, disulfiram, phenylbutazone or metronidazole.

61.E

The anatomical snuffbox is a triangular depression on the lateral side of the wrist. It is bounded medially by the tendon of the extensor pollicis brevis, and laterally by the tendons of the abductor pollicis longus and extensor pollicis brevis. It is accentuated by extending and abducting the thumb. The scaphoid bone and radial pulse can be palpated here.

62.D

Epinephrine has activity at all subtypes of adrenergic receptors, while norepinephrine has activity at alpha1, α-2, and β-1 receptors, but not at β-2 receptors. β-2 receptors found in blood vessels and are responsible for vasodilation. Because of this selectivity, **norepinephrine** (but not epinephrine) produces an increase in total peripheral resistance. Epinephrine also increases cerebral, muscle, and splanchic blood flow, and increases heart rate and cardiac output, while norepinephrine has little effect on these parameters.

63.D

Juvenile-onset diabetes mellitus, also known as insulin-dependent diabetes mellitus, results from a deficiency of insulin-secreting ß-cells in the pancreatic islets. Insulin was the first recombinant drug licensed for human use. Prior to production in bacteria, insulin to treat diabetics was obtained from the pancreas of pigs and cows.

64.E

Diphenoxylate induces an inhibition of intestinal peristalsis and is used as an antidiarrheal. It is chemically related to meperidine. The other opioids in the question are primarily used for pain relief.

65.E

Endothelin, a recently discovered peptide, is the most potent vasoconstrictor of those listed. AT II (not AT I) is a less potent vasoconstrictor. Prostacyclin (prostaglandin I_2) and nitric oxide are vasodilators, and heparin is an anticoagulant.

66.E

Sublimation involves channeling unacceptable impulses into acceptable avenues. **Altruism** is an unselfish interest in the welfare of others. The use of humor may indicate the ability to place one's existence in a larger perspective. These, along with suppression and anticipation, are considered mature defenses. **Projection** (attributing one's unacceptable thought to others) is more primitive and typical of an earlier period of life.

67.B

The frontal lobes are responsible for concentration, orientation, abstraction, language, judgment and problem-solving, and motor regulation. Of these, only language is localized to the left or right side. Reading comprehension, as well as object recognition, is a province of the dominant temporoparietal region.

68.E

Gamma IFN promotes the development of a population of helper T cells (Th-1) which mediate delayed-type hypersensitivity (DTH). Its production is enhanced by IL-12 and inhibited by IL-10. IL-12 is also mitogenic for T cells and NK cells. Moreover, the onset of DTH down-regulates IL-12 production.

69.A

Clostridium perfringes secretes an neurotoxin which produces paralysis by blocking acetylcholine release. Each of the other effects are mediated by endotoxin (LPS), which is also a polyclonal activator of B cells.

70.E; 71.A

Prosopagnosia is an inability to recognize faces which should be familiar. Facial recognition is a function of the nondominant parietal lobe. **Lethologica** is a temporary inability to remember a name or proper noun. **Agnosia** is an inability to recognize the significance of sensory impressions.

Synesthesia is a hallucination caused by another sensation (i.e., a sound is experienced as a smell). **Noesis** is a feeling that one has been chosen to lead and command others.

72.E; 73.B; 74.D

Linked subregions of the MHC complex on chromosome 6 in humans include the class I locus (containing A, B, and C loci), class II (containing DP, DQ, and DR loci), and class III (which encodes C2, C4, and the cytokines tumor necrosis factor and lymphotoxin). A person can make up to 12 HLA proteins (3 at class I and 3 at class II, from both chromosomes). Class I proteins bind the CD8 receptor of cytotoxic T cells, and class II proteins bind the CD4 receptor of helper T cells. Several diseases are correlated with HLA haplotypes; Reiter's syndrome and ankylosing spondylitis with B27, rheumatoid arthritis with DR4, multiple sclerosis with DR2, and myasthenia gravis with B8.

75.A

IL-2 and gamma IFN both stimulate CMI, while IL-4 is a B cell growth factor. Thus, the measles virus weakens CMI and delayed-type hypersensitivity, the most effective branch of immunity for handling viruses. Immunoglobulin levels are usually normal.

76.B

Resistance to erythromycin often involves plasmid-encoded enzymes which methylate the 23S rRNA. Plasmids also mediate resistance to penicillin and cephalosporin (through ß-lactamases), aminoglycosides (through enzymes which acetylate, adenylate, or phosphorylate), chloramphenicol (through acetylation), and to tetracycline and sulfonamides (through reduced uptake or increased export of drug). Quinolone resistance is primarily due to chromosomal mutations which alter the drug's target, bacterial DNA gyrase.

77.A

The sympathetic system is involved in «fight or flight» responses. It uses epinephrine and norepinephrine as its primary neurotransmitters. Functions include pupillary and bronchial dilation, increased heart rate and contractility, and decreased digestive processes.

78.E; 79.C

Phenobarbital is a sedative-hypnotic and anticonvulsant. Despite being a CNS depressant, phenobarbitol can produce excitability and hyperactivity in children. Primidone and diazepam are also anticonvulsants. **Dextroamphetamine** is a CNS stimulant and peripheral vasopressor; the mechanism by which it controls the symptoms of attention deficit disorder with hyperactivity is not well established. **Proproxyphene** is an opioid analgesic, and chlorpromazine is an antipsychotic.

80.C

Delirium is characterized by the sudden onset of disturbances of consciousness and changes in cognition which develop over a short time and tend to fluctuate during the day. Patients are often disoriented, have language abnormalities, and altered cognition and perception (hallucinations).

81.A

A long recognition sequence will cleave infrequently, yielding large DNA fragments which are convenient for long-range physical mapping. Cleavage to produce short fragments (as in B) would be less useful. Cleavage away from the recognition site provides no advantage in this case, nor does thermal instability. Mapping is possible with either blunt or overhanging (cohesive) ends.

82.A

The **mu** receptor is morphine-selective and mediates pain relief. **Kappa** receptors are specific for dynorphin, which mediates mild pain relief. Sigma receptors bind hallucinogenic opiates and ß endorphin. **Gamma** receptors mediate cognitive changes.

83.E; 84.C

Proprantheline is a quaternary ammonium anticholinergic which causes a decreased acid secretion and delayed gastric emptying by blocking vagal secretory and motor effects. **Misoprostol** is a synthetic prostaglandin E_1 analog with both antisecretory and mucosal protective properties. It is useful in the prevention of NSAID-induced gastric ulcers, but may be an abortifactant. **Ranitidine** and cimetidine are histamine H_2 receptor blockers; **omeprazole** is a proton pump blocker, and calcium carbonate is an antacid.

85.A

Relative risk is calculated for prospective (cohort) studies. It equals the incidence of a disorder among exposed individuals divided by the incidence of the disorder among unexposed individuals. An odds ratio is calculated for a retrospective (case-control) study.

86.E

Antibiotic resistance is a simple and frequently used way to identify and select recombinant DNA molecules. When incubated with the appropriate antibiotic, bacteria harboring nonrecombinant molecules are killed, whereas those with a resistance gene are spared. The other options in the question are either nonspecific or implausible.

87.C; 88.B; 89.A

Type I or immediate hypersensitivity reactions occur when IgE on mast cells and basophils is bound by an allergen, which results in the release of mediators (e.g., histamine) and the development of urticaria, rhinitis, etc. In **type II** or cytotoxic hypersensitivity, circulating blood elements are targeted and destroyed by IgG, IgM, phagocytes, and complement. **Type III** or hypersensitivity involves the deposition of immune complexes in the skin, joints, lungs, kidneys, and elsewhere; examples include serum sickness and systemic lupus erythematosus. **Type IV** delayed hypersensitivity is mediated by sensitized T cells; contact dermatitis is an example.

90.C

The pyramidal system contains axons of the corticonuclear tract (which go bilaterally to all brainstem motor nuclei except those controlling the lower facial muscles, which are contralateral) and axons of the corticospinal or pyramidal tract (which go to spinal motor nuclei; the lateral tract contains decussated fibers, while the ventral contains uncrossed fibers). The other tracts are found in the basal ganglia (nigrostriate), and midbrain (mamillotegmental and central tegmental).

USMLE step 1

BASIC MEDICAL SCIENCES

BOOK F TEST 2

ANSWERS

TEST 2

1.D

B. pertussis is an encapsulated gram-negative rod which causes whooping cough. It is noninvasive, and its toxins include dermatonecrosis toxin, tracheal cytotoxin, and pertussis toxin (which ADP-ribosylates an inhibitory G protein subunit). Up to 70% lymphocytes are seen on a peripheral blood smear. Although it can be prevented by immunization with killed organisms, incidence of the disease is rising, due in part to the fact that up to two-thirds of infants are underimmunized.

2.B

Cerebellar lesions may result in poor motor coordination, decreased cognitive function, poor timing of motor tasks, and increased reaction time to stimuli. The evidence in the question shows that the cerebellum is active in coordinating motor skills for sensory discrimination.

3.D

CEA and alpha-FP are two nonspecific markers for a variety of tumor types. They normally occur in higher levels in fetal tissue, and are more useful in following disease progression than in diagnosis. As a consequence of neoplastic transformation, many tumors acquire new antigens (tumor-associated antigens, TAAs), which may be involved in the occasional regression of tumors. In animal models, TAAs are highly specific when induced by a chemical, but often cross-react when induced by a virus.

4.C

Salmonella infection, a common cause of enterocolitis, generally yields stool samples containing neutrophils but no blood. In contrast, *Shigella, Campylobacter,* and *E. coli* tend to yield stool samples containing blood and neutrophils. *Escherichia* ferments lactose avidly, and *Vibrio* ferments lactose slowly; the other listed organisms are lactose nonfermenters. Among gram-negative enteric rods, only *Salmonella* and *Proteus* produce H_2S.

5.D; 6.E; 7.D

The **pineal** gland makes melatonin, which synchronizes internal rhythms. Signals from the suporachiasmatic nucleus of the hypothalamus cause the nocturnal elevation of melatonin. The pineal gland also contains corpora arenacea («brain sand»), visible in histological sections but of unknown significance. The **amygdala** is a collection of nuclei in the uncus of the temporal lobe which has connections with the hypothalamus, limbic and olfactory system, and brainstem.

8.E

There are no discrete post-translational mechanisms to alter immunoglobulin binding affinity. In addition to combinatorial association, junctional and insertional diversity, and somatic cell mutation, other mechanisms for generating antibody diversity include random assortment of heavy (H) and light (L) chains and the presence of multiple germ line V regions in both H and L chains.

9.A

The rapid onset of symptoms of food poisoning suggests an intoxication rather than an infection. *S. aureus* produces a heat- resistant enterotoxin which acts by stimulating the release of large amounts of interleukins-1 and -2. The other organisms would require several hours to produce symptoms.

10.D; 11.A; 12.B; 13.D

The dorsal columns (A), carry fibers for ipsilateral touch and pressure (the gracile tract for the lumbar and sacral areas, and the cuneate tract for the cervical and thoracic areas). A lesion of upper motoneurons (B) will produce ipsilateral spastic paralysis, while a lesion of the lower motoneurons (C) will produce ipsilateral flaccid paralysis. The spinothalamic tract (D) carries fibers for contralateral pain and thermal sensation. The ventral white commissure (E) carries bilateral pain and thermal fibers at each spinal cord level.

14.E

Upper motor neurons (UMNs) consist of nerve cells in the cerebral cortex which pass to lower motoneruons to initiate and regulate voluntary movements, especially skilled movements. Damage to UMNs results in «spastic paralysis» which affects the contralateral side if the lesion is above the pyramidal decussation and the ipsilateral side if the lesion is below. There are exaggerated myotatic reflexes, increased resistance to passive stretch (both of which are decreased in lower motoneuron (LMN) syndromes), and abnormal cutaneous reflexes (e.g., the Babinski sign). Muscle atrophy is pronounced in LMN lesions, but only slight in UMN lesions.

15.E

Rotavirus, a member of the reovirus family, is the most common cause of gastroenteritis in infants and young children. It replicates its segmented, double-stranded RNA genome in the small intestinal mucosa, damaging the transport mechanisms of ions, glucose, and water. **Norwalk** virus is a calcivirus with a single-stranded RNA genome of positive polarity; it causes diarrhea typically in young adults. ***V. parahaemolyticus*** is a diarrhea-causing bacteria found in seafood.

16.E

Gamma or fusiform neurons innervate intrafusal muscle fibers, and maintain muscle spindle sensitivity during contraction. **Alpha motoneurons** innervate extrafusal fibers of voluntary muscles; the term is synonymous with lower motor neuron. **Renshaw cells** mediate recurrent inhibition of alpha motoneurons. **Golgi tendon** organs are proprioceptive endings in tendons which decrease reflexive muscle contraction.

17.E

Several classes of antibiotics block bacterial protein synthesis and thus prevent the production of exotoxins. Aminoglycosides (e.g., streptomycin) and tetracyclines interact with the 30S ribosomal subunit. Chloramphenicol, erythromycin, and clindamycin interact with the 50S ribosomal subunit. In contrast, trimethoprim inhibits nucleotide synthesis by antagonizing the enzyme dihydrofolate reductase.

18.C

The **cerebellum** is divided horizontally into three lobes. Lesions of the anterior lobe which may result from the degeneration of Purkinje neurons in chronic alcoholics result in gait ataxia. Lesions of the posterior lobe result in an intention tremor. Lesions of the flocculonodular lobe result in balance disturbances manifested by poor coordination of the paravertebral muscles (truncal ataxia).

19.D

Estrogen tends to enhance immune responses, and this may contribute to the observation that women are affected more frequently than men by autoimmune disease. There is strong evidence suggesting that many autoimmune diseases result from a decreased number of suppressor T cells. Enhanced helper-cell function may be involved in drug-induced hemolytic anemias. Antibodies may form when sequestered antigens (such as myelin, lens proteins, and spermatozoa) are released into the circulation.

20.D; 21.B; 22.C

HAV is an enterovirus with an RNA genome. It is transmitted through the fecal-oral route and is not associated with chronic infection. **HBV** is an enveloped, partially double-stranded circular DNA virus which is transmitted through blood and sexual contact. **HCV** is an enveloped RNA virus which is clinically similar to HBV in terms of potential for chronic infection and predisposition to hepatocellular carcinoma) **HDV** (delta antigen) is a defective, single-stranded circular RNA virus which obtains its envelope from HBV and thus can only replicate in HBV-infected cells. **HEV** is a nonenveloped, single-stranded RNA virus implicated in water-borne epidemics outside the U.S.; chronic infection is rare, but there is a high fatality rate among pregnant women.

23.C

The visual fields are represented in the visual path such that nasal optic fibers cross, while temporal optic fibers remain ipsilateral, and all images are inverted. The left homonymous superior quadrant anopsia shown in the figure is explained by a right-sided lesion in the lower part (loop of Meyer) of the optic radiation (geniculocalcarine tract).

24.E; 25.B

In the diagram, «A» represents class II MHC, «B» represents the T-cell receptor, and «C» represents the CD4 protein, which stabilizes the interaction between the two cells. The HIV envelope protein gp120 has specificity for the CD4 receptor, which enables it to infect helper T cells. It is derived (along with gp41, which mediates fusion) from the 160 kD product of the env gene. p66 (reverse transcriptase) and p31 (integrase) are products of the pol gene. p24 corresponds to a major core protein. Each number corresponds to the protein's molecular weight in kilodaltons.

26.C

Poxviruses replicate in the cytoplasm and are not known to integrate into the host chromosome. Poxviruses are at least twice as large as other viruses. Molluscum contagiosum is characterized by small, wartlike lesions of the skin, and is especially seen in cases of immunodeficiency. Smallpox (caused by variola virus) was eradicated using a vaccine containing live, attenuated vaccinia virus.

27.A

The three layers of the cerebellar cortex include (from internal to external) the molecular layer (containing Purkinje dendritic trees as well as stellate and basket neurons), the Purkinje cell layer, and the granular layer. The Purkinje cells inhibit the cerebellar nuclei, and are themselves inhibited by stellate and basket cells. Granule cells excite the Purkinje, stellate, basket, and Golgi cells. Golgi cells inhibit the granule cells.

28.B

The tuberculin skin test is an example of delayed-type hypersensitivity; the reaction is due to recognition of the antigen by sensitized T cells. The positive test indicates a previous infection, not current disease. However, conversion of a negative to a positive test suggests a recent infection. Infected persons with immunosuppressive disorders may have a falsely negative test result.

29.D

Adenovirus and HPV are two viruses commonly implicated in carcinogenesis. Both express proteins which bind and inactivate tumor suppressor gene products. Specifically, proteins E1A (adenovirus) and E7 (HPV) bind RB1 (retinoblastoma), and proteins E1B (adenovirus) and E6 (HPV) bind p53.

30.E

HSV1, HSV2, EBV, CMV, and VZV are all DNA enveloped viruses belonging to the herpesvirus family. **HSV1** causes gingivostomatitis, herpes labialis, keratoconjunctivitis, and encephalitis. **HSV2** can produce genital herpes and aseptic meningitis. **EBV** causes infectious mononucleosis. In addition to causing congenital disease, **CMV** can produce retinal disease, mononucleosis, and pneumonia in immunocompromised patients. **VZV** causes chickenpox (primary) and shingles (recurrent).

31.D

The symptoms in this patient are consistent with an overdose of d-tubocurarine, a nondepolarizing (competitive) neuromuscular blocking agent. This agent blocks the action of acetylcholine at the nicotinic receptor site in skeletal muscle, producing paralysis which progresses from small to large muscle groups. This agent has no central nervous system activity. Hypotension, bronchospasm, and excessive secretions are due to d-tubocurarine-mediated release of histamine, ganglionic blockade, and decreased venous return. These effects can be antagonized with anticholinesterase agents.

32.C

The symptoms in this patient are consistent with an overdose of scopolamine, a competitive antagonist at cholinergic muscarinic receptors. Parasympathetic blockade results in decreased glandular secretion, paralysis of the pupillary sphincter and ciliary body, blockade of the vagus nerve. Tachycardia and inhibition of sweating can raise the body temperature. Other side effects include constipation and urinary hesitancy.

33.D; 34.E

DiGeorge's syndrome results from a defect in the third and fourth pharyngeal pouches, from which the thymus and parathyroid glands normally develop. Presenting symptoms include recurrent viral, fungal, or protozoal infections due to deficient T cells, and tetany due to hypocalcemia.

35.D

The trigeminal ganglia contain the primary neurons for touch sensations in the head. Touch and pressure are transmitted through the pontine trigeminal nucleus, while pain and thermal sensations are transmitted through the spinal trigeminal nucleus. Both pathways cross before synapsing in the VPM thalamic nucleus.

36.E

All paramyxoviruses (RSV, measles, mumps, parainfluenza) have fusion protein spikes which facilitate cellular entry. Mumps and parainfluenza viruses also contain neuramidase (NA) spikes, which hydrolyze the galactose-N- acetylneuraminic acid bonds of glycoproteins and glycolipids, which also aids entry. Measles, mumps, and parainfluenza viruses possess hemagglutinin (HA) spikes, which are recognized by surface receptors on RBCs. In mumps and parainfluenza viruses, the HA and NA are on the same spike.

37.A

Neural crest cells migrate throughout the embryo and differentiate into other cells, including: ganglion cells (dorsal root, sympathetic, parasympathetic, and sensory ganglion of CN V, VII, VIII, IX, and X), neurilemmal cells, melanocytes, leptomeninges (pia and arachnoid), and chromaffin cells of the adrenal medulla (not cortex).

38.A

A facultative parasite is an organism which has an optional free-living cycle. *Hartmanella, Naegleria,* and *Acanthamoeba* are all amoeba which are normally free-living (in freshwater lakes and soil), but may occasionally parasitize humans; the latter two genera are important causes of meningoencephalitis.

Strongyloides is a nematode which may exhibit a life-cycle which is either a homogonic (exclusively parasitic) or heterogonic (free-living and parasitic generations). *H. nana* is a tapeworm which requires a mammalian host (rodents or humans) to complete its lifecycle.

39.C; 40.A

Malaria is transmitted through the bite of a female Anopheles mosquito infected by any of four plasmodia: *P. vivax, P. ovale, P. malariae*, and *P. falciparum*. The latter organism is most serious, as it causes a high level of parasitemia and can affect RBCs of all ages (*P. vivax* infects mainly reticulocytes, and *P. malariae* infects only mature RBCs.) Banana-shaped gametocytes in RBCs are characteristic of *P. falciparum*. Malaria is treated with chloroquine. *T. cruzi*, transmitted by the bite of the reduviid bug, causes Chagas' disease; facial edema (chagoma or Romana's sign) indicates acute infection, and some patients develop cardiac arrhythmias and failure. The acute phase is treated with nifurtimox. *T. gambiense* causes sleeping sickness. *L. donovani* causes kala-azar, which affects organs of the reticulo-endothelial system.

41.B

Intermediate hosts of the tapeworm *D. latum* include fish and copepods. *Schistosoma* (blood fluke) species reproduce asexually in freshwater snails before free-swimming cercariae penetrate human skin. Other flukes with aquatic intermediate hosts include the lung fluke *P. westermani* (snails and crabs) and the liver fluke *Clonorchis sinensis* (snails and fish). Larvae of the nematode *Anisakis* can cause disease when ingested in raw seafood such as sushi. Larvae of the nematode *T. spiralis* are transmitted in undercooked meat, especially pork; in humans, the larvae grow in striated muscle cells.

42.D; 43.B.

Blastomyces is a dimorphic fungus which is endemic in North and Central America and transmitted through inhalation. Skin ulceration and the appearance of the yeast form at 37°C is characteristic. Other dimorphic fungi transmitted through inhalation include *Coccidioides* (endemic in the southwestern U.S.) and *Histoplasma* (endemic in the Ohio and Mississippi River valleys; it survives in macrophages). *Cryptococcus* exists only as a yeast (often in soil containing bird droppings) and can cause meningitis. *Aspergillis* exists only as a mold and causes pulmonary granulomas. The two agents above tend to be opportunistic, causing disease in persons with impaired immune systems.

44 .B

In the mixed-leukocyte reaction, stimulator lymphocytes from a potential donor are killed by irradiation and mixed with live responder lymphocytes from the recipient; the mixture is then cultured with labeled nucleotides. The greater the amount of DNA synthesis in responder cells, the more foreign are the class II MHC proteins in the donor cells. Thus, the low level of tritiated thymidine incorporation indicates that a kidney from person «D» is not likely to be rejected by person «C.»

45.B; 46.C; 47.D

Sensations for touch and pressure in the lower limb travel through the spinal ganglia to the gracile tract, and synapse in the dorsal column nuclei (B). Secondary neurons then cross in the medullary sensory decussation (C) and travel in the medial lemniscus (D) to the ventral posterior lateral (VPL) thalamic nucleus, which is the relay center for spinal sensations. The dorsolateral tract of Lissauer and the spinothalamic tract conduct pain and thermal sensation from spinal levels, while the trigeminothalamic tract conducts cranial pain and thermal sensation. The ventral posterior medial (VPM) thalamic nuclei is a relay center for cranial sensations.

48.E

In this assay, antigens (Ag) and antibodies (Ab) diffuse through the gel and form precipitin lines when complexes are formed at the proper concentration. Ag2 contains some but not all of the epitopes as Ag3 (as would be the case with a homologous Ag from another mammal.) Ab not binding Ag2 continue to diffuse, and combine with Ag3, forming a spur. This spur always points to the Ag containing fewer recognized epitopes.

49.C; 50.D; 51.B

Common variable hypogammaglobulinemia is an acquired disorder of B cells, in which immunoglobulin synthesis is impaired. ***Wiskott-Aldrich syndrome*** is characterized by repeated pyogenic infection, thrombocytopenia, and eczema in the first year of life; T cell immunity is variable. **Hereditary angioedema** is an autosomal dominant condition; in the absence of its inhibitor, C1 esterase continues to act upon C4 to produce vasoactive kinins. **Chronic granulomatous disease** involves a deficiency of phagocytic killing of organisms due to a lack of NADPH oxidase. **Bruton's agammaglobulinemia** is X-linked and is characterized by a virtual absence of B cells due to a lack of a tyrosine kinase signal protein.

52.E; 53.E; 54.B

The gram stain separates bacteria into gram-positive (blue) and gram-negative (red) on the basis of cell wall properties. Gram-positive cell walls have thicker, multilayered peptidoglycan and contain teichoic acids while lacking LPS (endotoxin) and having less lipid. A capsule may be present on either type of cell wall. To perform the stain, crystal violet is added to a slide with fixed bacteria cells. Next, iodine (a mordant) is added to form a complex with crystal violet. Next, acetone is added, which extracts the blue dye complex from the lipid-rich, thinner gram-negative cell walls; the gram-positive bacteria remain blue. Finally, safranin stains the decolorized gram- negative cells red. *Neisseria* appear as gram-positive diplococci.

55.E

Glutamate, an excitatory neurotransmitter, is used in about 60% of the brain's synapses. Ten percent of synapses are GABAergic, and only 2% use dopamine, norepinephrine, serotonin, or acetylcholine.

56.A

A viral RNA with positive polarity is identical to messenger RNA. Because this genome is directly infective, the virus requires no transcription and hence encodes no polymerase. Poliovirus is a single-stranded, nonsegmented virus with positive polarity. Examples of viruses with other characteristics include paramyxoviruses («B»), orthomyxoviruses («C»), retroviruses («D») and reoviruses («E»).

57.B

Dementia is a syndrome characterized by multiple impairments in cognitive function without impaired levels of consciousness (as in delirium). The incidence of dementia increases with age; 20% of 80 year-olds are severely demented. Fifty to 60% of dementias are of the Alzheimer's type, another 15-30% are due to infarcts (vascular). About 15% of persons with dementia have illnesses which may be reversible.

58.C

Plasmin is activated by factor XIa or kallikrien; it degrades fibrin. Urokinase (from the kidney tubules) and streptokinase (from bacteria) both potentiate the action of plasmin. Heparin is a glycosaminoglycan which serves as a cofactor for antithrombin III, an inhibitor of several factors (IIa, IXa, Xa, XIa, XIIa, and XIIIa) in the coagulation cascade.

59.A

In organs receiving dual autonomic innervation, the effects of the two divisions are usually opposed. Sites at which sympathetic tone predominates include: arterioles, veins, cardiac ventricle, and sweat glands. At the first three sites, transmission is via adrenergic receptors; sweat glands are cholingeric. Sites at which parasympathetic tone predominates include: cardiac atrium and SA node, iris, ciliary muscle, gastrointestinal tract, urinary bladder, and salivary gland. Transmission at each of these sites is through cholingeric receptors.

60.E

The Fahraeus-Linquist effect states that the apparent viscosity of blood increases as the caliber of the blood vessel increases. Pouseille's law states that Q = (ΔPπr4)/(8Lh), where Q = flow, ΔP = pressure gradient, r = radius, L = length, and h = apparent viscosity.

61.D

In 1990, there were over 93,000 accidental deaths in the U.S.; half of these involved motor vehicles. Thirteen percent were due to falls and 7% were due to poisoning. Other causes, in decreasing order, included drowning, fires, suffocation, and firearms.

62.C

Stretch receptors are located in the wall of the internal carotid artery near its origin; these mechanoreceptors discharge at a rate directly proportional to arterial pressure. Occlusion of the common carotid arteries will cause a decreased pressure at these receptors, initiating a reflex increase in sympathetic discharge and a reflex decrease in vagal discharge, resulting in an increased blood pressure and heart rate.

63.C

Accidents account for nearly half of the deaths between the ages of 1 and 24. Death from accidents are most frequent on Saturdays and in the summer. Reasons for a higher rural accident death rate may include different occupational conditions and availability of trauma care.

64.D

Starling's law of the capillary states that J = Kf[(Pc-Pi) - ø(πc-πi)] - L, where J is net outward flow of capillary fluid, Kf is the filtration coefficient, Pc and Pi are capillary and interstitial hydrostatic pressures, πc and πi are capillary and interstitial colloid osmotic pressures, and L is lymph flow.

65.A; 66.E

In the U.S., the suicide rate has remained fairly constant, at 12.5 per 100,000. Almost 95% of all people who commit suicide are mentally ill; 80% are depressed, 10% are schizophrenic, and 5% are demented or delirious; another 25% are alcohol dependent or personality disordered. Over half see a physician in the month before the attempt. Suicide is the third leading cause of death from age 15-24 (behind accidents and homicide). Suicide rates increase with age. Women attempt suicide 4 times more often, but men complete suicide 3 times more often. Persons with borderline and histrionic personality disorders tend to attempt suicide most often, while persons with antisocial personality disorder tend to complete suicide most often.

67.A; 68.B; 69.D

The patient's low pH indicates an acidosis; this can be explained by the loss of bicarbonate (due to diarrhea), which is compensated by a decrease in $PaCO_2$. As a rule of thumb, in metabolic derangements, the blood gas values ($PaCO_2$ and bicarbonbate) are deviated in the same direction as the pH deviation, while in respiratory derangements, the blood gas values are deviated in the opposite direction.

The anion gap equals sodium - (chloride + bicarbonate), and is normally 12 mEq/L. Conditions which account for a low anion gap include increased unmeasured cations (lithium, calcium, immunoglobulins, etc.), or decreased anions (decreased albumin, or decreased charge on albumin as in acidemia). A high anion gap could be explained by an increase in unmeasured anions (lactate, ketones), uremia, or toxic organic acids (methanol, ethylene glycol). Intravenous bicarbonate will help to replace the losses and will offset the acidosis. Hyperventilation and IV lactate would exacerbate the problem, and 100% oxygen is not indicated. Although an anticholinergic agent might decrease the episodes of diarrhea, it would improve the acidosis only slowly, and would not address the etiology of the diarrhea.

70.D

Medicaid is designed for low income persons and is funded federally and by states. Medicaid is a program for those eligible for Social Security, and is federally funded. HMOs are private organizations available to anyone who is willing to prepay for services. About 15% of Americans have no health insurance.

71.B; 72.C; 73.E

Hodgkin's lymphoma (HL) is characterized by the presence of Reed-Sternberg (RS) cells (arrow) admixed with a heterogeneous lymphocytic population. RS cells show prominent, mirror-image nucleoli with a clear halo around them. RS-like cells have been found in several benign and malignant lymphoid pathologies. Most patients with HL present with lymphadenopathy. The nodes are firm or rubbery. If necrosis of the lymph node occurs, they may be soft. The homogeneous surface of a cut lymph node produce the «fish flesh» appearance (gray-white tissue). Spleen is involved in one third of the cases at the time of diagnosis, although in most patients the spleen is affected at autopsy. The liver is rarely affected at the time of diagnoses but at autopsy the liver is involved in 2/3 of the patients. The bone marrow can be affected by discrete foci of fibrotic tumor. As the disease progresses, destruction with an osteolytic appearance on radiologic examination is common. A multifocal infiltration of malignant plasma cells in the bone marrow is seen in multiple myeloma.

74.C

Common side effects of lithium use are: polyuria/polydipsia (50%), leukocytosis (30-45%), Muscular weakness (33%), GI disturbance (30%), T wave inversion (20-30%), weight gain (25%), hypothyroidism (3-30%), and tremor (4%). Uncommon side effects include acne, psoriasis, edema, and cardiac dysrhythmia. Lithium toxicity at high serum levels may be fatal.

75.A

The bones of the calvaria (cranial vault) include the paired frontal and parietal, and the squamous part of the occipital bone. These (as well the maxilla and part of the mandible) undergo intramembranous ossification. The sphenoid, ethmoid, and petrous temporal bones, as well as the base of the occipital bone, undergo endochondral ossification.

76.B

Osteoporosis (OP) is characterized by a reduction in bone mass per unit of bone volume. About 25% of women over age 60 have radiographically detectable OP, making it the most common bone disorder seen clinically. Postmenopausal estrogen deficiency is a key factor in the development of OP. **Osteomalacia** is characterized by inadequate mineralization of newly formed bone matrix. **Osteomyelitis** is an infectious bone inflammation. **Osteopetrosis** (marble bone disease) is characterized by abnormally dense bone due to hypofunctional osteoclasts. **Ankylosing spondylitis** is an inflammatory arthropathy of the vertebral column.

77.D

PTH is the primary regulator of serum calcium; it increases calcium levels by promoting bone resorption, and also through action on the kidney and gut. **Calcitonin** (made by the thyroid parafollicular cells) lowers serum calcium by inhibiting bone resorption. Vitamin D3 (cholecalciferol) is produced in the skin from 7-dehydrocholesterol through the action of sunlight; it is dihydroxylated (at the 25 position in the liver and the 1 position in the kidneys) to its active form, 1,25- OH-2-vitamin D3. It enhances gut absorption of calcium, phosphate, and magnesium. Estrogens,
as well as, insulin, androgen, growth hormone, and thyroid hormone promote bone formation.

78.B

HMG-CoA reductase is the critical regulatory enzyme of cholesterol biosynthesis. The NADPH-dependent reaction occurs in the endoplasmic reticulum. It is inhibited by the drug lovastatin, which inhibits de novo cholesterol synthesis and upregulates the number of LDL receptors.

79.C

Vitamins A, D, E, and K are fat-soluble, isoprenoid compounds which (like steroids) are composed of activated five-carbon units. Vitamin C is water soluble and contains a furan ring.

80.A; 81.E; 82.D

Deficient dietary intake of water soluble vitamins can result in disease. **Folic acid** (pteroylmonglutamic acid) is needed for nucleic acid synthesis and erythrocyte maturation; a deficiency can result in megaloblastic anemia. **Thiamine** (vitamin B_1) is involved in oxidative decarboxylation reactions; deficiency (beri-beri) has arisen when polished rice is the major caloric source, and can involve peripheral neuropathy, Wernicke's encephalopathy, muscle weakness, edema, and cardiac failure. **Riboflavin** (vitamin B_2) is a cofactor for enzymes (such as pyruvate dehydrogenase) which catalyze electron transfers; clinical signs of deficiency include cheilosis, angular stomatitis, seborrheic dermatitis, and interstitial keratitis of the cornea. **Biotin** is a coenzyme for carboxylation reactions; deficiency can result in dermatitis, muscle weakness, depression, and memory impairment.

83.E

Cytosolic proteins are marked for degradation by ubiquitination of lysine groups. Oxidation of methylene groups to ketones also favors proteolysis. Essential amino acids include arg, his, ile, leu, phe, thr, val, lys, met, and trp; the latter three can become deficient in vegetarian diets. Nonessential amino acids can be synthesized by the body and are not expressily required in the diet; these include glu, gln, asp, asn, ala, gly, pro, ser, tyr, and cys (a mnemonic «GYPSY CANED Q» comes from the one-letter abbreviations). Positive nitrogen balance prevails pregnant women and growing children, while negative nitrogen balance occurs in malnutrition and disease.

84.C

Pyridoxal phosphate (the coenzyme form of vitamin B6) and tetrahydrofolate (THF) are both involved in one-carbon metabolism. SAM performs biological methylation reaction such as the conversion of homocysteine to methionine. Ascorbic acid (vitamin C) is required for the hydroxylation of lysine and proline residues in collagen.

85.D

Serotonin and nicotinamide nucleotides (NAD+) are both derived from tryptophan. Phenylalanine may be converted to tyrosine, which gives rise to catecholamines (dopamine, epinephrine,...etc), thyroid hormones, and melanins. Histidine is decarboxylated to form histamine. Glutamate undergoes decarboxylation to form GABA.

86.C

The formation of PRA, an activated sugar phosphate, from 5-a-D-phosphoribosyl-1-pyrophosphate (PRPP) is the first committed step in the de novo synthesis of purines. After a series of reactions, inosine monophosphate, with its characteristic purine double-ring structure, is produced.

87.D

The lac operon consists of three linked structural genes that encode enzymes of lactose utilization. The repressor binds the operator site, thereby blocking transcription. The repressor also has a binding site for an inducer (such as lactose or allolactose); binding the inducer inactivates the repressor by decreasing its affinity for DNA. Once the repressor is removed, RNA polymerase may bind at the initiation site, and the genes are expressed.

88.A

The adrenergic receptor is a classic model of a seven TMD receptor. During synthesis, the N-terminus is anchored to the membrane by a hydrophobic sequence, which serves as a start signal for translocation. The second hydrophobic sequence serves as a translocation stop signal. The remaining six signal regions alternate between start- and stop-sequences until the entire protein is generated, with the C-terminus located intracellularly. Cleavage of the first signal peptide yields a new N-terminus which is located on the external side of the cell. The receptor loops (between TMDs 2-3, 4-5, and 6-7) are also located externally.

89.E

Deoxynucleotides (eg., dGDP) are all synthesized from their corresponding nucleotide diphosphate (eg., GDP) by the same enzyme, rNDP reductase, which replaces the 2-hydroxyl group of ribose with a hydrogen atom. Once formed, three of the diphosphates (dATP, dGDP, and dCDP) are converted directly to triphosphates by nucleoside diphosphokinase. In contrast, dUMP (formed from dCMP or dUTP) is converted to dTMP by thymidylate synthase.

90.B

Fatty acid synthesis occurs in the cytosol. Parts of the urea cycle occur in both the mitochondria and cytosol. The other listed processes occur predominantly in the mitochondria.

USMLE step 1

BASIC MEDICAL SCIENCES

BOOK F TEST 3

ANSWERS

1.B

IL-1 and TNF alpha are produced mainly by macrophages. Many of the other interleukins, including IL-2, IL-4, IL-5, IL-6, and IL-12, are produced by helper T lymphocytes.

2.B

SCID involves an absence of both B and T cells, due to a defect in early stem cell differentiation. It may be X-linked (which often involves an impaired IL-2 receptor), or autosomal (which may involve an absence of class II MHC). Toxin neutralization is mediated via antibodies, and would be defective in SCID patients. The other aspects of natural immunity are less impaired.

3.B; 4.E; 5.A

Glycoprotein spikes («A») are usually specified by the viral genome, and mediate binding to specific receptors on target cells. The lipoprotein viral envelope («B») contains lipid from the host cell membrane, acquired by the virus during budding. The capsid («D») contains the nucleic acid («E») within the core («C»). The capsid contains the principle antigenic epitopes in nonenveloped viruses. Infective virus disappears during the eclipse period. Thereafter, the multiplication cycle proceeds by replicating the viral genome, synthesizing viral proteins, and forming progeny viral particles.

6.E

Nitroglycerin relaxes vascular smooth muscle and dilates both arterial and venous beds. This promotes peripheral pooling of blood and decreases venous return. Arterial pressure and myocardial oxygen consumption are also reduced.

7.B

Dapsone is primarily used in the treatment of leprosy. Protocols for tuberculosis treatment often include combinations of the following drugs: isoniazid, rifampin, ethambutol, streptomycin, and pyrazinamide.

8.C

The two obligations for persons entering the sick role are to seek professional help and to comply with the prescribed regimen.

9.C; 10.A

Oligonucleotide mutagenesis is performed by constructing a DNA sequence which is nearly complementary to a target DNA sequence. By hybridizing these sequences and extending the synthetic primer, the newly polymerized DNA molecule will differ from the parent at the chosen site. Linker scanning mutagenesis involves the generation of a random set of deletion mutants. DNase I protection mapping (footprinting) can identify protein-DNA binding sites, as unbound DNA is enzymatically fragmented. A mobility shift assay is a method to detect DNA binding proteins in crude protein extracts. ELISA offers a way to quantify antigens or antibodies.

37.C; 38.B; 39.A; 40.E

Collagenous colitis is characterized by chronic or episodic watery diarrhea and the presence of a distinct collagenous band beneath the colonic surface epithelium. The mean age is 60 years and it affects women more than men in a ratio 4:1. This disease is considered a form of autoimmune disorder. Differential diagnosis includes ulcerative colitis and Crohn's disease when the collagenous band is thin or discontinuous.

41.E; 42.B

In this population, 1000 will be infected and 9000 will not be infected. Use the sensitivity and specificity figures to fill in the table.

	test +	**test -**	**total**
Known +	900	100	1000
Known -	1800	7200	9000
Total	2700	7300	

The number of false positives is 1800 (20% of the true negatives). The positive predictive value is 900/2700 and the negative predictive value is 7200/7300.

43.D

In negative reinforcement, an unpleasant stimulus is removed when a desired behavior occurs. In positive reinforcement, a desired behavior is rewarded with something pleasant.

44.C

Panic disorder has a lifetime prevalance of up to 3%, and is equally common in men and women. It is characterized by the recurrent, abrupt onset of symptoms such as palpitations, sweating, trembling, dyspnea, nausea, dizziness, and fear of losing control. Sodium lactate often induces panic attacks in patients with panic disorder, but there is a 28% false-positive rate.

45.A; 46.D

Classically, osteoblasts are assigned the role of bone formation and osteoclasts (multinucleated cells derived from monocytes) are assigned the role of bone degradation. However, osteoblasts respond to bone-resorbing hormones by secreting proteases such as tissue plasminogen activator (tPA) and collagenase. Bone matrix, produced by osteoblasts, is about half organic (type I collagen, glycoproteins, and proteoglycans), and half inorganic (mainly calcium hydroxyapatite [= Ca10(PO4)6(OH)2]). The adult skeleton consists of 80% compact (dense) bone and 20% trabecular (cancellous) bone.

47.A; 48.C

The median nerve enters the wrist by passing through the carpal tunnel, behind the flexor retinaculum (which attaches laterally to the scaphoid and trapezium and medially to the pisiform and hamate bones.) Carpal tunnel syndrome results from compression of the nerve within this tunnel. Typically, symptoms consist of pain or tingling along the lateral three and one half fingers and weakness of the thenar muscles, which corresponds to the distribution of the median nerve. In question 48, option A describes a radial nerve palsy, and option D describes an ulnar nerve palsy.

49.D

Hydrochlorothiazide is a diuretic and antihypertensive which enhances renal excretion of Na+, Cl-, and water to decrease intravascular volume. The site of action is primarily the distal nephron. Adverse effects can include hypokalemia, hyperuricemia, metabolic alkalosis, hyponatremia, hypercalcemia, and hyperglycemia.

50.C

The cytochrome P450 (CYP) enzyme superfamily (mixed function oxidases) are found in the smooth endoplasmic reticulum of the liver and other organs. In addition to metabolizing drugs and foreign chemicals, CYPs also perform endogenous functions such as adrenal and gonadal steroidogenesis, hydroxylation of cholesterol and vitamin D metabolites, and synthesis of prostacyclin and thromboxane. Metabolism of epinephrine is carried out by monoamine oxidase (MAO) and flavin-containing monooxygenase (FMO).

51.A

Isolation involves the separation of an unpleasant idea from its associated feeling. Undoing is an impulse to perform an action which is the reverse of an unwanted idea or feeling, such as repeatedly locking and unlocking a door to make sure it is locked.

52.D

The interstitial cells of Leydig produce testosterone, while the Sertoli cells of the seminiferous tubules produce primary spermatocytes. The prostate gland and seminal vesicles supply the fluid component of semen.

53.B

Chordae tendinae prevent the atrioventricular valves from flopping back into the atria during the heart cycle. They are anchored to ventricular papillary muscles and are not part of the conduction system. Chordae tendinae are not present on the aortic and pulmonic valves.

54.E

Ethical consultations are used to make patient-oriented decisions, and are becoming increasingly utilized. Once it is decided to perform an autopsy, the decision of who will perform it does not normally warrant an ethics consultation.

55.A

FSH induces an increase in cyclic AMP in the Sertoli cells, which stimulates production of ABP. LH activates the Leydig cells to produce testosterone.

56.E

The superior mesenteric artery arises directly from the abdominal aorta, just distal to the celiac trunk.

57.E; 58.D; 59.D

This patient suffers of **celiac sprue**. It is characterized by a flattened mucosa with marked atrophy and distortion of the superficial glandular epithelium. A heavy chronic inflammatory infiltration including plasma cells, lymphocytes, macrophages, eosinophils and mast cells is also present. The columnar epithelium shows reactive atypia and several mitotic figures. The hallmark histopathological findings are a flat small intestinal mucosa with blunting or disappearance of villi, damaged epithelial cells on the mucosal surface and increased cellularity of the lamina propria but not of the deeper layers.

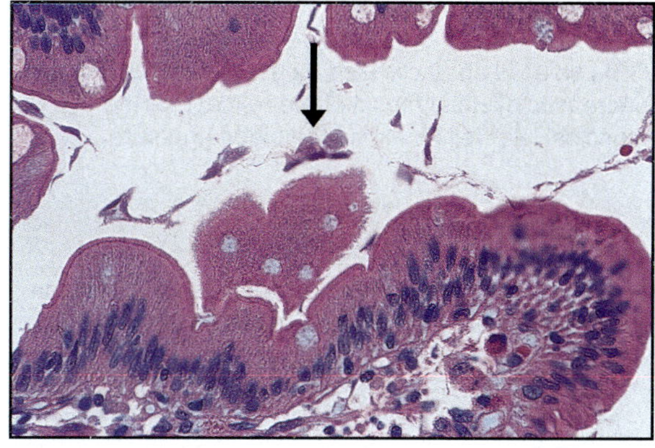

Figure 46 (3.60)

60.C; 61.B; 62.A

The picture (figure 46) shows **giardiasis** of the duodenum with several parasitic forms showing a sickle-shaped profile, some sitting on the epithelial brush border. One form shows a sagittal section with display of characteristic two nuclei . The mechanism of diarrhea and malabsorption of giardiasis is not well known. There is not evidence of exo or endotoxins production. Mucosal injury by the parasite (reduction in villus height and increased lymphocytes in the lamina propria) and the bacterial overgrowth have been described.

63.E; 64.A

The microphotograph shows a cluster of malignant cells with a very high nuclear/cytoplasmic ratio, large hyperchromatic nuclei with distinct nucleoli. In this case, a good reference for size evaluation is the use of the red blood cells present in the field. If red cells have an approximate diameter of 7 um, the tumor cells show approximately 6 to 8 times this size (40-50 um diameter). The presence of blood in sputum also correlates with tumor diathesis. Other syndromes associated with lung carcinoma are inappropriate secretion of anti-diuretic hormone (SIADH), hypercalcemia, acromegaly, Myasthenia Gravis-like syndrome...etc.

65.B

REM sleep is characterized by paralysis and decreased skeletal muscle tone (except for the eye muscles), as well as increased blood pressure.

66.A

Learned helplessness has been used as a model for major depression. Animals become listless and despondent.

67.D

The anterior fascial compartment of the forearm typically consists of eight muscles arranged in four layers. The most superficial muscles are the pronator teres, flexor carpi radialis, flexor carpi ulnaris, and the palmaris longus (which is absent in about 13% of individuals.) The second layer includes the flexor digitorum superficialis. The third layer contains the flexor pollicis longus and the flexor digitorum profundus. The fourth and deepest layer contains the pronator quadratus. The anconeus is found in the posterior fascial compartment of the forearm.

68.B

The principle of double effect explains the relationship between the intended act (providing relief) and the unintended consequence (the hastening of death). **Consequentialism** considers only the ultimate consequences of an act. **Utilitarianism** is the idea of providing the «greatest good for the greatest number.» **Deontology** refers generally to ethics and moral obligation. **Teleology** is similar to determinism.

69.C

Compared to skeletal muscle, smooth muscle has smaller fibers, contracts more slowly and more powerfully, and has twice as much actin and tropomyosin but four times less myosin. Unlike skeletal muscle, actin and myosin form an inactive complex independent of ATPase activity. The resting membrane potential is about 30 mV less negative than skeletal muscle, and the resistance is ten times greater, indicating the presence of fewer ion channels.

70.C

The septum transversum is the primordium of the central tendon of the diaphragm. The diaphragm also derives from the pleuroperitoneal membranes, dorsal esophageal mesentery, and the body wall. The septum primum and septum secundum are found in the developing heart.

71.A

Physiostigmine is an anticholinesterase and as such potentiates cholinergic activity, such as glandular secretion. The other listed signs and symptoms are characteristic of a cholinergic blockade.

72.A

Nifedipine (procardia) is a calcium channel blocker useful in the treatment of both classical and vasospastic angina. It dilates the coronary arteries and reduces oxygen utilization. It has been associated with the development of congestive heart failure in some individuals.

73.B

Cortisol is hypersecreted in depression. This is the basis for an abnormal dexamethasone test (DST) in 50% of patients who have major depression with melancholia. The DST also may be positive in pregnancy, schizophrenia, many systemic illnesses, and 5% of the normal population.

74.A; 75.E

MCV is derived by dividing the Hct by the RBC count; the normal range is 80-90 μm^3. The MCHC is derived by dividing the [Hb] by the Hct; the normal range is 25-30 picograms (1 pg = 10-12 g). The Hct is the percentage of blood composed of RBC; the normal range is 35-42% for women and 40-46% for men. The [Hb] is measured in g/dL (g/%); the normal range is 12-14 g/% for women and 14-17 g/% for men.

76.A

The gluteus maximus extends and laterally rotates the hip. The gluteus medius, gluteus minimus, and piriformis are all abductors of the hip. The gracilis is primarily a flexor of the knee.

77.C

Administering intravenous sodium amobarbitol may result in a temporary improvement in patients with conversion disorder (formerly known as hysteria), psychosis, and anxiety. However, it results in increased cognitive impairment in patients with delirium or dementia.

78.E

The left anterior descending (LAD), or left anterior interventricular artery, is the most common site of infarction. The right coronary artery and circumflex branch of the left coronary artery are second and third most frequent, respectively. The coronary sinus drains venous blood to the right atrium.

79.C; 80.B; 81.E

Selectivity for adrenergic receptors is fundamental to many drugs. Agonists at the alpha receptor include phenylephrine (alpha-1) and clonidine (alpha-2). Antagonists at the alpha receptor include prazosin (alpha-1), yohimbine (alpha-2), and phenoxybenzamine (nonselective). Agonists at the beta receptor include dobutamine (beta-1), terbutaline (beta-2), and isoproterenol (nonselective). Antagonists at the beta receptor include metoprolol (beta-1), butoxamine (beta-2), and propranolol (nonselective).

82.A

The WCST requires cognitive flexibility to decipher the changing patterns. Individuals with isolated prefrontal lesions often score well on IQ tests but poorly on the WCST.

83.D

The long bones cease to contribute substantially to erythropoiesis after the age of twenty. The axial skeleton (vertebrae, sternum, ribs) is the primary site of RBC production throughout the adult lifespan.

84.D

In the case of portal hypertension, blood flow through systemic and portal anastomoses is enhanced to help decrease portal pressure. The paraumbilical veins anastomose with the iliac veins, (leading to caput medusae) the gastric with the azygous veins (leading to esophageal varices), and the superior rectal with the middle and inferior rectal veins (leading to hemorrhoids).

85.E

Patients with OCD have been found to have smaller caudate nuclei with an increased local metabolic rate. Abnormalities in the temporal cortex have been found in patients with bipolar disorder. Hypoplasia of the cerebellar vermal lobules has been observed in autistic patients. Enlarged lateral ventricles and wide cortical sulci have been demonstrated in patients with schizophrenia and depression.

86.C; 87.B; 88.E

On this graph, menstruation occurs at the left side of the Y-axis, and ovulation occurs at the midpoint, between the follicular and luteal phases. FSH (D) induces the early development of the follicle, and declines prior to ovulation. Estrogens (A) are secreted by the follicle and later the corpus luteum and induce endometrial changes. Ovulation is induced by a surge of LH (C). Progesterone (B), secreted by the corpus luteum, peaks after ovulation and also helps to thicken the endometrium. If fertilization occurs, hCG (E - not shown), made from the embryo-placental unit, rescues the corpus luteum from degeneration.

89.B

Though the course of Alzheimer's is variable, the typical course is a change in personality, then mood, then intellectual skills, then a loss of recent memory, then social and hygienic skills, then language skills, and then bladder and bowel control.

90.A

In the extrinsic coagulation pathway, factor VII is cleaved to VIIa (plasma proconvertin) by factor III (tissue thromboplastin, released from damaged endothelium). Factor VIIa cleaves factor X to Xa (prothrombinase). In the final common pathway, factor Xa cleaves thrombinogen to thrombin (factor II). Thrombin converts fibrinogen to a fibrin monomer, which polymerizes spontaneously and is stabilized by factor XIIIa (which is also activated by thrombin).

USMLE step 1

BASIC MEDICAL SCIENCES

BOOK F TEST 4

ANSWERS

1.D

Most oncogenes are mutated forms of normal genes (proto-oncogenes). Proto-oncogenes have diverse biochemical properties, including a) protein kinase (*abl, src, trk*); b) GTPase (*H-ras, N-ras*); c) DNA-binding (*myc*); d) steroid receptor (*erb A*), and e) ß-chain of platelet-derived growth factor (*sis*).

2.B

The energies associated with the listed interactions are inversely dependent on the distance between the molecules. A dipole occurs when an uncharged molecule has a polarized electron distribution such that one end has a slightly negative charge and one end has a slightly positive charge. The strength of molecular interactions (in descending order) are as follows (r=radius). 1) charge-charge (1/r); 2) charge-dipole (1/r2); 3) dipole-dipole (1/r3); 4) charge-induced dipole (1/r4); 5) dipole-induced dipole (1/r5); 6) dispersion (mutual synchronization of fluctuating charges; 1/r6) and 7) hydrogen bonds (fixed bond length, about 0.3 nm).

3.E

The Henderson-Hasselbalch equation states pH = pKa + log {[A-]/[HA]}, where [HA] is the concentration of undissociated acid (proton donor), and [A-] is the concentration of the conjugate base (proton acceptor). Here, (3.86) + log (10) = 4.86.

4.D

The pI is the point when the average charge on the substance being titrated is zero. At point «B» (the inflection point representing pKa1), the amino acid is doubly protonated; at point «E» (pKa2), the amino acid is doubly unprotonated. Between these two points («D»), the amino group is protonated (+ charge) and the carboxyl group is unprotonated (- charge), for a net molecular charge of zero.

5.C

High-energy phosphate compounds drive many thermodynamically unfavorable reactions through coupling. The free energy change (ΔGo', kJ/mol) for the hydrolysis of PEP is -62; for BPG = -49; for CP = -43; for pyrophosphate = -33; for ATP and ADP = -31; and for AMP to adenosine + Pi = -14.

6.E

People of low socioeconomic status tend to postpone or avoid seeking the help of medical professionals, which contributes to their tendency to be relatively sicker and to stay longer when admitted to the hospital.

7.D

When $p < .05$, the results are statistically significant to the 95% confidence level, and the null hypothesis should be rejected.

8.E

Chi squared assesses the significance between proportions (frequencies). T-test analyzes the difference between means of two samples, while ANOVA tests differences between means of more than two samples. Correlation tests the mutual relation between two continuous variables, while regression analysis tests the relation between many measures.

9.B

Ego functions include reality testing and perceptions, intellect, motor and sensory functions, interpersonal relationships, and mood. The **superego** is comparable to conscience. Both the ego and superego have conscious, unconscious, and preconscious components. The **id** is an unconscious store of primitive drives.

10.C

Passive aggression is an ego defence mechanism that involves translating one's angry feelings into quiet defiances.

11.D; 12.C; 13.E

Kaposi's sarcoma is commonly seen in association with AIDS. Histologically, this tumor shows jagged, thin-walled, dilated vascular spaces in the epidermis. There is extravasation of red blood cells and diffuse hemosiderin deposits admixed with interstitial infiltration by inflammatory cells. This tumor is derived from endothelial cells. It is associated with AIDS patients who have declining the immunity. The nodules can spread to the lungs and other tissues or organs.

14.A; 15.A

Breast cancer is the most common cancer in women in the United States. Currently 7% of the American women may be expected to develop this disease by the age of 70 years. It is uncommon before the age of 35 years and there is a strong association a family history of breast cancer. Early menarche, late menopause, and older age at first-term pregnancy, all increase the risk of this disease. Oophorectomy before age 35, but not after, dramatically *lowers* the risk of breast cancer. The histology of the biopsy shows an intraductal or invasive carcinoma, with a cartwheel or cribriform pattern of cellular growth. The solid tumor growth is interrupted by several small circular spaces of vayiring size. Stromal invasion, fibroblastic proliferation and formation of duct-like structures also are present.

16.C

The energy charge of a cell describes the capacity of the cell to carry out ATP-driven reactions, and is defined as ([ATP] + 0.5[ADP])/([ATP] + [ADP] + [AMP]). In this example, the energy charge is (2+2) / (2+4+2) = 4/8 = 0.5. Most healthy cells function at energy charges of about 0.9.

17.D

G_1 cyclins function in performing phosphorylation reactions which signal a commitment to cell division.

18.E

Proline is a cyclic amino acid which disrupts regular alpha helical structures.

19.E

The side chain of lysine consists of four carbons and an amino group; the side chain of leucine consists of four carbon groups. Seven amino acids have ionizable side chains (in increasing order of pKa): Asp, Glu, His, Cys, Lys, Tyr, and Asp. Proteins absorb UV light at a peak of 280 nm due to the aromatic side chains in Phe, Tyr, and Trp. Basic amino acids (His, Lys, and Arg) act as proton acceptors.

20.A

Peptide bonds are metastable; hydrolysis is thermodynamically favored (ΔGo' = -10 kJ/mol) but occurs very slowly at physiological temperature and pH.

21.B

About 68% of scores fall within one standard deviation (S.D.) of the mean. About 95% of scores fall within two S.D. (so 2.5% are above and 2.5 % are below). About 99.7% of scores fall within three S.D.

22.C

Schizophrenia has a lifetime prevalence of 1.5% and an incidence of 0.5%. It is about equal in incidence between men and women and is seen in all cultures.

There is a strong genetic influence (concordance approaches 50% in monozygous twins). it most commonly occurs under the age of 35. Psychotic symptoms, deterioration from previous levels of functioning in such areas as work, social relations, and self care, for a period of more than 6 months. Flat or grossly inappropriate affect is common.

23.D

Night terrors (pavor nocturnus) occur during slow wave sleep (NREM stage 3/4); typically there is no recollection of the event in the morning. Night terrors may develop into sleepwalking. Nightmares occur during REM sleep.

24.A

According to Kubler-Ross, the stages in the process of dying are denial, anger, bargaining, depression, and acceptance. They may be experienced in any order.

25.B

Seven percent of all births are premature. The U.S. ranks 20th in infant mortality (0.9%). Caesarean births have increased in recent decades to nearly 1/5 of all deliveries. Major depression affects 5-10% of women after childbirth; only 0.2% of these women develop postpartum psychosis. Primitive reflexes are typically present at birth.

26. E

Antinuclear antibodies are tested by immunofluorescent (IF) techniques or by ELISA. The figure shows the «speckled» pattern of IF with a granular appearance of the nuclei and negative staining of the nucleoli. These antibodies are specific for ribonucleoproteins and histones. However, the presence of these antibodies is not specific for lupus erythematosus, and it can be seen in several autoimmune disorders. Approximately 5% of the elderly population may have these antibodies in low titer in the absence of clinical disease.

27.C; 28.C; 29.B (see figure 47)

Burkitt's lymphoma is a small non-cleaved cell lymphoma . Even though the histological appearance of the African (endemic) and the non-endemic Burkitt's lymphomas are identical, they have some clinical and virologic differences. The figure shows a tumor with a monotonous population of 10-25 um diameter cells with round or oval nuclei containing two to five prominent nucleoli. Several mitotic figures are present. Several pale-staining benign tissue macrophages (arrow) are typically present. These macrophages, when seen at low power magnification, impart to the tumor a «starry sky» appearance. The Endemic Burkitt Lymphoma is endemic in Africa and New Guinea. The Epstein-Barr viral genome is present in 95% of the cases. The Sporadic Burkitt Lymphoma harbors the Epstein-Barr viral genom in only 15% of the cases. The most common sites of involvement in the Endemic type, include the jaw bones. Burkitt and Burkitt-like lymphomas are the most common lymphomas in AIDS patients. More than 50% of the cases long-term survival can be expected with the present methods of treatment.

30.E; 31.A; 32.D

The figure shows extensive hepatic necrosis which is more evident around the central vein (right arrow); a portal space (left arrow) is also seen. Toxic doses of acetaminophen (between 15 to 25 g) cause centrilobular necrosis that may extend to entire lobules. Simultaneous alcohol ingestion may have a synergistic effect. A concomitant evidence of renal, lung and myocardial damage may be present. This toxicity is attributable to the formation of toxic metabolites (i.e. n-acetylimidoquinone) which are normally detoxified by glutathione. With extreme overdoses, the glutathione is depleted and the reactive metabolites bind to other vital hepatic proteins resulting in cell injury. An overdose of 10 g or more in an adult may result in the potentially fatal hepatic necrosis. Administration of N-acetylcysteine, which contains

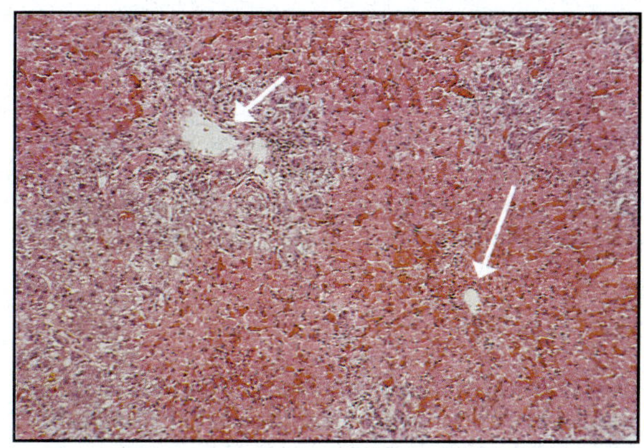

Figure 47 (4.30)

sulfhydryl froups to which the toxic metabolite can bind, can be lifesaving.

33.B

From the start codon AUG, the sequence is read in triplets until the first in-frame stop codon (UAG) is encountered. Here, fifteen bases (corresponding to 5 amino acids) are read. Other stop codons include UAA (out of frame here) and UGA (in frame but downstream).

34.E

The insulin gene contains four exons (signal, B-chain, C-chain, and A-chain). It is translated as pre-proinsulin, which is a random coil. The leader sequence helps the polypeptide move through the endoplasmic reticulum (ER) membrane, and then it is cleaved, leaving proinsulin. In the ER, the polypeptide is folded, and disulfide bonds (one in the A-chain and two interchain) are formed. After passing through the Golgi apparatus, the C-chain (C peptide) is cleaved. Insulin in its native conformation is localized centrally within the granule, while C-peptide molecules are peripheral.

35.C

The thermodynamics of protein folding is described by the free energy equation, $\Delta G = \Delta H - T\Delta S$ (where G = free energy, H = enthalpy, T = temperature, and S = entropy). Protein folding is favorable (i.e., ΔG is negative). Although folding decreases the entropy of the system (making the reaction less favorable), this is compensated for by effects which decrease the enthalpy (intramolecular side group interactions and the hydrophobic effect).

36.A

An example of operant conditioning is seen in an athlete who trains hard in anticipation of winning a trophy. In classical conditioning, a reflex response follows a stimulus.

37.E

One-word speech and standing are normal developmental milestones for one year. Rolling over, sitting, and walking typically begin at 5, 7, and 15 months respectively.

38.B

Wave types, from fastest to slowest, are beta, alpha, theta, and delta. Beta occurs during attentiveness, alpha during relaxation, and delta in deep sleep. Focal delta and theta waves may indicate pathology.

39.D

The mini-mental state test is a standardized screening tool with a maximum score of 30. It tests orientation, registration and recall, attention and calculation, and language skills (such as reading, writing, copying, and following commands). Abstract reasoning may be tested separately, for example by asking a subject to interpret a metaphor.

40.A; 41.B

Schizoid personality disorder affects up to 5% of the general population; such individuals tend to be quiet loners with a restricted range of emotions. Unlike avoidant personality disorder, these individuals are socially detached by preference rather than due to feelings of inadequacy, inferiority, or fear of rejection. Schizotypal personality disorder has a lifetime prevalence of 3%. It involves a pattern of social deficits, perceptual distortions, and eccentric behavior.

42.B; 43.A; 44.D

The figure shows two very atypical endocervical cells with a high nuclear/cytoplasmic ratio, clumped chromatin, distinct nucleoli and vacuoles in their cytoplasm. These cells are most consistent with an adenocarcinoma of the cervix. An endocervical curetting with endometrial biopsy in the diagnosis work up should be performed. Squamous carcinoma cells do not show this morphology with cytoplasmic vacuolation. This tumor is associated with adenocarcinoma *in situ* and are frequently infected with HPV types 16 and 18.

45.B; 46.C; 47.B

The pattern of netlike fluorescence seen in this figure is characteristic of intercellular deposits of IgG specific for desmosome proteins. This reactivity is more evident in the sites with acantholysis, and it is mostly seen in cases of pemphigus vulgaris. The lesion is large, easily ruptured blister that leaves extensive denuded or crusted areas. Without corticosteroid and/or immunosuppressive treatment, the disease is progressive and usually fatal.

48.B

Primary structure refers to the linear amino acid sequence (and any disulfide bonds) present in a protein. **Secondary structure** refers to spatial arrangements assumed by local regions of polypeptides; common examples include alpha helices (right-handed, 3.6 residues per turn) and flat ß-sheets (antiparallel chains have opposite N-to-C directions). **Tertiary structure** refers to the way that secondary structure elements are folded to yield an overall three-dimensional structure. **Quaternary structure** applies to proteins with multiple subunits (e.g., hemoglobin with two alpha and two beta chains).

49.C

Ligases (like pyruvate carboxylase, which forms oxaloacetate from pyruvate and carbon dioxide) catalyze reactions in which two molecules are joined. **Lyases** (e.g. pyruvate decarboxylase) usually involve reactions at double bonds. **Hydrolases** (e.g., carboxypeptidase) involve cleavage with the addition of water. **Transferases** (e.g., glucokinase) catalyze the transfer of functional groups between molecules. **Isomerases** (e.g., malate isomerase) catalyze cis-trans intramolecular rearrangement.

50.D

Reversible inhibitors bind noncovalently to the active site (competitive) or to a secondary site (noncompetitive) on the enzyme. A competitive inhibitor is a false enzyme substrate; it increases the apparent K_M but does not affect the V_{max}. A noncompetitive inhibitor decreases the enzyme's catalytic efficiency; it decreases the V_{max} but does not affect the K_M.

51.D

Trypsin and chymotrypsin are examples of serine proteases. The serine hydroxyl group is highly reactive due to the orientation of aspartic acid, histidine, and serine (the catalytic triad) in the active site. This reactivity acts as a charge transfer system during catalysis.

52.A

The Golgi apparatus is a site where numerous protein modifications occur, including glycosylation reactions. Alpha-mannosidase (which removes sugar residues) is a marker for the Golgi apparatus.

53.E; 54.A; 55.B

The figure shows a renal glomerulus with a linear pattern of fluorescence indicating the presence of anti-glomerular basement membrane antibodies. This antibody reactivity is typical of Goodpasture's syndrome which is a triad of diffuse alveolar hemorrhage, glomerular nephritis and a circulating cytotoxic autoantibody to basement membrane. Histologically, erythrocytes and hemosiderin-laden macrophages fill the airspaces. The alveolar septa are mildly thickened with interstitial fibrosis and hyperplasia of type II pneumocytes. Patients present hemoptysis, dyspnea, weakness and mild anemia. Evidence of glomerulonephritis follows the pulmonary manifestations. Corticosteroids, cytotoxic drugs and plasmapheresis can increase the 2-year survival only to 50 percent.

56.C; 57.E

Arnold Chiari malformation is the most common of the Chiari's malformations (type II). The major components are: (1) displacement of the cerebellar tonsils into the cervical canal; (2) Z kink distortion of the medulla at the cervicomedullary junction; and (3) a small, shallow posterior fossa with enlarged foramen magnum. This malformation is almost always associated with both hydrocephalus and spinal dysraphism. The picture shows dysraphism. The hydrocephalus is not always significant. The brain stem and cerebellum are compacted into a shallow, bowl-shaped posterior fossa with a low positioned tentorium. It is associated with meningomyeloce. It causes hydrocephalus, through obstruction of the foramina of Magendie and Luschka.

58.C; 59.C

The picture shows benign columnar, ciliated cells, representing normal bronchial epithelium. The presence of cilia in bronchial cells is not observed in malignant cells. The finding of bronchial epithelial cells indicates that the sputum sample is optimal for evaluation. Another important element for good sample quality is the presence of alveolar macrophages.

60.E, 61.B

The double reciprocal plot shows the variation of reaction velocity with substrate concentration according to the Michaelis-Menton equation, $V = V_{max}[S] /([S] + Ks)$, where Ks is a dissociation equilibrium constant for the enzyme-substrate complex. In the plot, $1/V_{max}$ occurs at the Y intercept («B»). KM is associated with the binding strength of enzyme to substrate; $-1/K_M = 1/[S]$ at the X intercept («A»).

62.B

There are five multiprotein complexes in the respiratory assembly, with progressively greater standard reduction potentials (E'0, in parentheses). Complex I shuttles electrons from NADH (-0.32) to FMN (-0.3) to an iron-sulfur (Fe-S) center; complex II shuttles electrons from FAD (-0.22) to an Fe-S center to cytochrome b560; both complex I and II converge at CoQ (+0.04). Complex III carries electrons from CoQ to cyt b (0.07) to cyt c1 (0.23) to cyt c (0.25); complex IV (cytochrome oxidase) carries electrons from cyt a (0.29) to cyt a3 (0.55) to molecular oxygen (0.82). Complex V is the F0F1 ATP synthase. Three reactions have ΔGo' values greater than the 30.5 kJ/mol for ATP hydrolysis; FMN to CoQ, cyt b to cyt c1, and cyt a to O2.

63.A

Oxidation reactions involve a loss of electrons, while reduction reactions involve a gain of electrons. Cytochrome oxidase is the enzyme complex which transfers electrons from cytochrome a to O_2, a reaction which is inhibited by carbon monoxide and cyanide.

64.E

The P/O ratio is the number of ATP molecules synthesized per pair of electrons carried through electron transport. Due to their entry positions in the electron transport chain, the P/O of NADH is generally accepted as 3.0, and the P/O of FADH is 2.0. Thus, 3(3) + 2(2) = 13 ATP molecules. The actual value is likely to be less than this ideal value due to the less-than-perfect efficiency of the system.

65.A; 66.C

HbS (sickle-cell hemoglobin) results from a transition mutation in the 6th codon of the gene for the ß hemoglobin chain, where the normal GAG sequence is present as GTG. This leads to a missense mutation in the amino acid sequence, as a valine is substituted for a glutamine. Clinically, after a time delay, deoxygenated hemoglobin molecules tend to aggregate or «sickle,» forming polymers by a double nucleation mechanism. The autosomal trait (the alpha locus is on chromosome 16 and the ß locus is on chromosome 11) offers heterozygote carriers some resistance to malaria. The aliphatic side chain on valine is less polar than the acidic side chain on glutamine, hence HbS («C») runs slower on a gel than HbA («A»). Carriers («B») express HbA and HbS codominantly.

67.D

Using open-ended questions during interviewing allows the patient to describe her complaint in her own words. Items B and C are closed-ended questions which can be answered briefly. Items A and E might be interpreted as being confrontational or judgmental.

68.C

Erikson's stages are as follows: trust vs mistrust (age 0-1), autonomy vs shame and doubt (age 1-3), initiative vs guilt (age 3-5), industry vs inferiority (age 6-11), and identity vs diffusion (age 11-20). Adulthood is marked by intimacy vs isolation, generativity vs stagnation, then ego integrity vs despair.

69.B

The mean is the arithmetic average, median is the middle number of a sequentially arranged set, and mode is the most commonly appearing number. In this example, the mean, median, and mode are 4.3, 4, and 3, respectively.

70.E

To generalize, the southern states tend to have the lowest per capita income (Mississippi ranks last with a mean yearly income just over $18,000). These states are also underserved by doctors.

71.E; 72.A; 73.D

When confronted by this type of problem, it is helpful to construct a table like this one:

	test +	**test -**	**total**
known +	90	10	100
known -	30	70	100
total	120	80	

The sensitivity of a test is the percentage of known positives who test positive. In this case 90/100 = 90%. The specificity of a test is the percentage of known negatives who test negative - in this case 70/100 = 70%. The positive predictive value (chance that a positive test result is accurate) is calculated by dividing the known positives by the total number of positive tests - in this case 90/120 = 75%. Also, the negative predictive value here is 70/80 = 87.5%

74.A

Extinction occurs when the frequency of a behavior (going to class) diminishes as rewards for it (exam scores) diminish. **Habituation** is a decrease in a reflex response to a repeated stimulus. **Sensitization** is an exaggerated response to a repeated stimulus.

75.C

Examples of projective tests include the Rorschach ink blot test, thematic apperception test, sentence completion, word-association, and the draw-a-person test. They attempt to reveal unconscious influences upon personality and behavior.

76.D

Somatization disorder is characterized by multiple, medically unexplained symptoms, typically in young women. If two of the following seven symptoms are positive in the context of an appropriate history, somatization disorder is 90% likely: dyspnea, dysmenorrhea, vomiting, amnesia, bloating, lump in the throat, and painful extremities.

77.B; 78.B

Adult polycystic kidney disease causes end-stage renal failure in 8-10 % of the patients. Fifteen percent of the patients develop brain aneurysm. One third of the patients develop liver cysts. It is inherited as an autosomal dominant trait. The cysts are as large as 5 cm in diameter. Patients present symptoms by the fourth decade, with flank masses and passage of blood clots in the urine. Azotemia is common in half of the cases and progresses to uremia in several years.

79.D; 80.E

Erythema multiform appears to be a hypersensitive response to certain infections and drugs. This disorder is a prototype of a cytotoxic reaction pattern with extensive epithelial cell degeneration and death. A diversity of lesions are present, including maculas, papules, vesicles, and bullae, with characteristic target lesions consisting of red maculae or papulae with pale vesicular eroded centers.

81.E

This is a lymph node with reactive lymphoid follicles displaying enlarged follicular centers. The anti-CD20 reactivity confirms that this is a polyclonal population and that there is no fusion of the follicular structures, which favors a benign process. The CD20 marker is specific for B cells, in contrast to the CD3 marker which recognizes T cells. B lymphocytes proliferate in the response to liposaccharide.

82.B; 83.C

Wilms Tumor is a malignant mixed tumor of the kidney composed of mesenchymal and epithelial embryonal elements. It is one of the most common solid tumors in children, and usually presents before the age of 4 years. Histologically, the tumor has metanephric blastema (small ovoid cells), immature stroma (undifferentiated spindle cells) and immature epithelial elements (small tubular structures). Most children present with a large abdominal mass accompanied by pain and occassionally with intestinal obstruction.

84.E; 85.B

The figure shows several areas of alveolar fibrosis with fibrous thickening of the small lung vessels. This case corresponds to a patient with progressive systemic sclerosis (PSS) with pulmonary hypertension. PSS is associated with a variety of immunologic abnormalities, changes in the systemic microvasculature, and excessive fibrosis. Virtually all organs may be involved in PSS.

86.D

Axis I of the DSM IV (Fourth Diagnostic and Statistical Manual of the American Psychiatric Association) encompasses clinical disorders. Axis II encompasses personality disorders and mental retardation. Axis III involves general medical conditions. Axis IV involves psychosocial and environmental problems (such as health care access, housing and economic problems). Axis V involves a global assessment of functioning scale (based on 100 points).

87.C; 88.E

Bipolar disorder classically features alternating depressive and manic episodes. The disorder begins with a depressive episode in 70% of patients, but 10-

20% have only manic episodes. It has a higher incidence in the higher socioeconomic status group. Treatment typically includes an antimanic agent (lithium) and an antidepressant (such as amitriptyline), but not antipsychotics. With treatment, only 15% recover completely. 75% have relapses or a partial remission, and 10% receive no benefit from therapy. A more favorable prognosis is associated with female gender, advanced age at onset, and a short duration of episodes.

89.B

Addiction includes tolerance needing higher doses to produce the same effects, and significant withdrawal symptoms such as seizures and tremors.

90.A

Incidence is the total number of new cases in a population during a specified period of time. Prevalence is the number of cases at any given time. For a common pathogen which is quickly cured but may infect numerous times, the total number of cases in a year will be greater than the number of cases at a given time.

USMLE step 1

BASIC MEDICAL SCIENCES

BOOK F TEST 5

ANSWERS

1.B

Herpes simplex virus has the unique property of being tropic for the central nervous system, which might make it useful in the hypothetical scenario presented. HIV is tropic for CD4+ T cells. The other viruses are able to infect a greater variety of cell types.

2.B

The cranial nerves (CN) III, VII, IX, and X carry parasympathetic fibers. The oculomotor nerve and its ciliary ganglion carry fibers for pupillary constriction and accommodation. The facial nerve and its geniculate ganglion, and the glossopharyngeal nerve and its otic ganglion carry fibers involved in glandular secretion, specifically, the lacrimal, submandibular, sublingual, nasal, and palatal for CN VII, and parotid for CN IX. The vagus nerve and its dorsal vagal nucleus carry fibers to smooth muscle and glands in the pharynx, larynx, and thoracic and abdominal viscera.

3.C

The structure shown in the figure is an IgA dimer with a J (joining) chain (dark bar) and a secretory component (arc). The J chain is present in IgA dimers and IgM pentamers. Only the secretory IgA molecule has a secretory component.

4.B

Saccharomyces cerevisiae (baker's yeast) is a eukaryotic organism useful in genetic cloning because of its rapid growth and relatively small genome. *B. hermsii, E. coli*, and *A. israelii* are all prokaryotic organisms. *C. immitis* is eukaryotic but currently has no use in recombinant technology.

5.E

The trochlear nerve innervates the superior oblique muscle and produces inward rotation and downward and lateral movement of the contralateral eye.

6.C; 7.A; 8.D

Complement is a series of serum proteins which are activated in cascade fashion. C3b receptors are present on the surface of many phagocytes, hence C3b is important in opsonization (enhancing phagocyosis). C5a, along with C3a and C4a, are anaphylatoxins which cause mast cell degranulation. C5a and the C567 complex attract neutrophils (chemotaxis). The membrane attack complex (MAC), which inserts into cell membranes, is comprised of C5b6789. Decay-accelerating factor (DAF) prevents the formation of the MAC by destabilizing C3 convertase and C5 convertase.

9.A

Increased viral diversity is not correlated with progression of AIDS; in fact, the accumulation rate of mutant RNAs has been correlated with a slower progression of the disease. This may be due to selective pressure placed on viral subtypes by a functioning immune system.

10.A

Astrocytes proliferate in response to injury, forming a «glial scar». The other listed CNS components typically degenerate following an injury.

11.D

Protein synthesis proceeds from the amino terminus to the carboxyl terminus. In DNA synthesis, the newly-replicated strand grows from the 5' to 3' direction (but the parental template is read from 3' to 5').

12.A

Ribosomal RNA comprises about 80% of the RNA found in a cell. Transfer RNA comprises about 15%. Messenger RNA, which contains the most variable sequences and has the highest turnover rate, comprises the remaining 5%.

13.B

About 68% of scores fall within one standard deviation (S.D.) of the mean. About 95% of scores fall within two S.D. (so 2.5% are above and 2.5 % are below). About 99.7% of scores fall within three S.D.

14.B

Schizophrenia has a lifetime prevalence of 1.5% and an incidence of 0.5%. It is about equal in incidence between men and women and is seen in all cultures. There is a strong genetic influence (concordance approaches 50% in monozygous twins). It is best treated with antipsychotic drugs. It most commonly occurs under the age of 35.

15.D

MRSA is a frequent problem in hospital or nursing home patients. The treatment of choice is **vancomycin**. This antibiotic is a mixture of glycopeptides. and inhibits the synthesis of bacterial cell wall phospholipids as well as peptidoglycan polymers. Aminoglycosides and third generation cepholosporins are useful in the treatment of gram negative bacteria, specially *P. areuginosa*. **Clindamycin** is effective against *S. aureus* sensible to methicillin.

16.B

Apolipoproteins are polypeptide markers which are important in the trafficking of lipid. Lipoproteins become more dense as they acquire a greater protein composition. Apo A-1 and A-2, and D are found only on HDL. Apo B-48 is found only on chylomicrons; it is lost upon processing to VLDL. Apo C-2, C-3, and E are found on chylomicrons, VLDL, and HDL.

17.B; 18.A; 19.A

Arachidonic acid (AraA) is produced by the action of phospholipase A2 on membrane lipids. AraA is metabolized by cyclooxygenase (CO) to a pathway which produces prostaglandins and thromboxane; CO is the major target of aspirin and most NSAIDS. AraA is also metabolized by lipoxygenase (LO) to a pathway producing 5-HPETE and leukotrienes.

20.B; 21.A; 22.E

The eosin-positive specific granules of eosinophils contain at least four major cytotoxic proteins, including eosinophil cationic protein, eosinophil protein X, eosinophil peroxidase, and major basic protein. Basophilic binding of IgE results in the release of histamine, which is involved in hypersensitivity reactions. The «drumstick» appendage on neutrophils represents a condensed X chromosome.

23.A

The **lag phase** (A) is a time of vigorous metabolic activity but few mitoses. In the **log phase** (B), the bacterial cells divide rapidly. The **stationary phase** (C) is a time of balanced cell division and cell death (due to scarce nutrients or toxic products). The number of bacterial cells declines during the **death phase** (D).

24.D

Kluver-Bucy syndrome is related to morphological changes in the limbic system. The visual agnosia results from damage to the temporal lobes, while hypersexuality, attentiveness, orality, and docility result from lesions to the amygdala. Memory loss is seen in Korsakoff's syndrome.

25.A

CD («cluster determinants») are functional markers on leukocytes. The binding of CD40 (on B cells) and p39 (on T cells) stimulates B cell activation. The binding of CD28 (on T cells) to B7 (on B cells) stimulates T cells; exposure to anti-CD28 antibodies has been shown to induce anergy.

26.D

The most common cause of meningitis in infants is Group B Streptococcus (*S. agalactiae*), followed by *E. coli.* In children, common causes include *Haemophilus influenzae*, followed by *Neisseria meningitides* and *Streptococcus pneumoniae*. In adults, *S. pneumoniae* is the most common cause, followed by *N. meningitides*. Staphylococcus species (*S. aureus, S. epidermidis*) may cause meningitis in trauma patients. *Listeria monocytogenes* and *Klebsiella pneumoniae* are less common causes which can strike any age group.

27.D

The left hemisphere is dominant for language in 97% of people (99% of right-handers and 60% of left handers).

28.E; 29.D

Streptococci are gram-positive, tend to grow in chains, and are catalase-negative (as opposed to *Staphylococci*). *Streptococci* are divided into different groups based on the pattern of hemolysis when grown on blood agar and antibiotic sensitivity. Alpha hemolytic streptococci form a green zone around their colonies due to incomplete lysis of red blood cells; an optochin disk further divides them into *S. pneumoniae* (sensitive) and *S. viridans* (resistant). Beta hemolytic streptococci leave a clear zone around their colonies; a bacitracin disk further divides them into Group A Strep (e.g., *S. pyogenes*, sensitive) and Group B Strep (e.g., *S. agalactiae*, resistant). Colonies which produce no hemolysis (gamma) and are soluble in bile are classified as Group D Strep (e.g., *S. faecalis* and *S. bovis*).

30.E

Mitochondrial DNA is predominantly inherited maternally, which has made it useful in evolutionary studies. It has a high mutation rate and does not recombine. There are two codons (UGA and AUA) which are translated differently than nuclear sequences. In addition, mitochondria have only 22 tRNAs, while over 40 species are available for cytoplasmic translation.

31.A

According to Kubler-Ross, the stages in the process of dying are denial, anger, bargaining, depression, and acceptance. They may be experienced in any order.

32.B

Seven percent of all births are premature. The U.S. ranks 20th in infant mortality (0.9%). Cesarean births have increased in recent decades to nearly 1/5 of all deliveries. Major depression affects 5-10% of women after childbirth; only 0.2% of these women develop postpartum psychosis. Primitive reflexes are typically present at birth.

33.E

People of low socioeconomic status tend to postpone or avoid seeking the help of medical professionals, which contributes to their tendency to be relatively sicker and to stay longer when admitted to the hospital.

34.D; 35.B

Histrionic personality disorder involves a pattern of excessive emotionality and attention-seeking. **Narcissistic personality disorder** involves a pattern of grandiose behavior, a need for admiration, and a lack of empathy; the process of aging is also handled very poorly.

36.E

Iodine is the most effective skin antiseptic used in medicine. Chlorine, mercury, silver, and hydrogen peroxide are also oxidizing agents which interact with sulfhydryl groups in proteins. **Ethanol** causes membrane disorganization and denatures proteins. Detergents and phenols also disrupt membranes, but the latter is seldom used today due to toxicity.

37.D; 38.B

A classic example of receptor-mediated endocytosis is seen in the low-density lipoprotein (LDL) receptor. After LDL is bound, the receptor-ligand complex is internalized and directed to primary endosomes. These then fuse with secondary endosomes (where the receptor-ligand complex is dissociated), which subsequently fuse with the trans Golgi network (TGN). The TGN directs the LDL receptor back to the cell surface and LDL to a degradative pathway of primary and secondary lysosomes. The movement and fusion of these subcellular compartments is dependent upon cytoskeletal interactions, particularly microtubules. Colchicine (used clinically to treat gout) is an inhibitor of microtubule assembly and polymerization.

39.A

The homeobox genes are important in pattern formation in limb development. The sequences are highly conserved evolutionarily, and have been studied extensively in Drosophila.

40.C

Individuals with this mutation develop the **William's syndrome**. They are mentally retarded but can read. They tend to have narrow aortas, short stature, fine bones, and elfin facial appearances. Mutations in a recently identified gene for performing spatial tasks makes these individuals unable to put together jigsaw puzzles.

41.A

The rabies virus is found most commonly in bats and skunks. It is rarely transmitted to humans (only 0-5 times per year) by contact with secretions of infected animals.

42.A

Conduction velocity (CV) is directly related to nerve fiber diameter, which is largely determined by the degree of myelination. Cutaneous touch and pressure are transmitted through small myelinated fibers, with a CV of 35-75 m/s. Fast pain travels through smaller myelinated fibers with a slower CV. Slow pain travels through unmyelinated fibers. Temperature travels through unmyelinated fibers and the smaller myelinated fibers. Afferent impulses from primary muscle spindles tend to travel the fastest, as they are transmitted by large myelinated fibers.

43 E; 44.B; 45.C

Interleukin 1 activates lymphocytes, neutrophils, fibroblasts, and other cell types. It induces the expression of IL-2, and is an endogenous pyrogen. IL-2 is an important stimulator of T cells. IL-4 enhances B-cell growth and may promote hypersensitivity. IL-5 promotes B-cell differentiation and stimulates IgA and eosinophil production. IL-6 is involved in inflammatory reactions. IL-8 promotes chemotaxis of many cell types.

46.D; 47.E; 48.C

In community acquired pneumonias, half are bacterial (typical); viral, mycoplasmal, and chlamydial pneumonias account for about 15% each. **Mycoplasmas** are small, wall-less organisms; the cold agglutinins are IgM autoantibodies against type O RBCs that agglutinate at 40°C but not 37°C. **Chlamydia** pneumoniae is an obligate intracellular bacteria which is transmitted by respiratory droplets. **Legionnaire's disease** accounts for about 8% of pneumonias, and is caused by *Legionella pneumophila*; outbreaks are often associated with environmental water sources. Q fever is caused by ***Coxiella burnetii***, a rickettsial organism; its reservoirs include farm animals and raw milk, and it is transmitted by inhalation of aerosol.

49.D

The production of multiple clones of T cells is stimulated by anti-CD3, PHA, ConA, and superantigens such as enterotoxin. Polyclonal activation of B cells occurs upon stimulation with anti-immunoglobulin, *S. aureus* (Cowan strain 1) and Epstein-Barr virus. PWM stimulates T and B cells.

50.C

There are three species of eukaryotic RNA polymerase. RNA polymerase I transcribes ribosomal RNA (forming the 5.8S, 18S, and 28S rRNAs). RNA polymerase II transcribes messenger RNA and small nuclear ribonucleoprotein particles (snRNPs). RNA polymerase III transcribes all transfer RNA genes as well as 5S rRNA. Prokaryotes have a single form of RNA polymerase. None of these polymerases has an inherent ligase activity. Retroviral reverse transcriptase uses an RNA template to manufacture DNA.

51.B

Here, the total number of cases (**prevalence**) will exceed the number of new cases in a given time (**incidence**).

52.A

Major depression and mania are distributed equally among the social classes.

53.E

Regression is a return to an earlier stage of functioning (such as acting childishly). It is common during stressful situations like being hospitalized.

54.B

The **ego** includes reality testing and perceptions, intellect, motor and sensory functions, interpersonal relationships, and mood. The **superego** is comparable to conscience. Both the ego and superego have conscious, unconscious, and preconscious components. The **id** is an unconscious store of primitive drives.

55.A

In steroid hormone synthesis, the initial step (cholesterol to pregnenolone) and the final steps (which produce aldosterone, cortisol, and testosterone) all occur in the mitochondrion. Many of the intervening steps (such as pregnenolone to progesterone) occur in the endoplasmic reticulum.

56.D

The transcription-coupled process of mismatch repair has been found to be defective in patients with hereditary nonpolyposis colorectal cancer. This has been linked to an increased rate of spontaneous mutation of microsatellite DNA sequences.

57.E

The P_{50} is the partial pressure of oxygen at which the carrier protein is half saturated. Myoglobin has a higher O_2 affinity and thus a lower P_{50} than does hemoglobin. The oxygen affinity of hemoglobin is increased by increasing the pH (Bohr effect), decreasing the pCO_2, decreasing the concentration of 2,3-DPG, and decreasing the temperature.

58.B

In the erythrocyte, much of the carbon dioxide combines with water to produce carbonic acid, most of which is converted to bicarbonate (70% of the total CO_2 in venous blood). About 23% is bound to hemoglobin as Hb-CO_2, and about 7% remains in gaseous form.

59.D

Some viruses make multiple types of mRNAs from a single piece of nucleic acid by «shifting the reading frame» in which codons are interpreted.

60.A

The *C.diphtheria* vaccine (like the vaccine for *Clostridium tetani*) is a toxoid (i.e., exotoxin treated with formaldehyde to eliminate functionality while preserving antigenicity). Vaccines using killed organisms as antigens include those for *S. typhi, V. cholerae*, and *Y. pestis*; the vaccine against *B. pertussis* may either use killed organisms or be acellular. The vaccine against tuberculosis utilizes live *M. bovis* organisms.

61.A

The locus ceruleus at the floor of the fourth ventricle contains cell bodies of over half the NE neurons in the CNS. The raphe nuclei contain serotonin. Dopamine is found in the basal ganglia, mesocortical-mesolimbic tract, and the tuberoinfundibular tract. The nucleus basalis is an area of acetylcholine concentration.

62.A

Given the child's HLA markers, the mother's haplotype is A1, B8, DR4 / A11, B27, DR4. The child inherited the first set from her, and another set (A5, B44, DR6) from someone other than Mr. R, who lacks two of the three markers.

63.E

Endotoxins are cell wall components of gram-negative bacteria, while exotoxins are produced by either gram-positive or gram-negative bacteria. Exotoxins are much more toxic than are endotoxins (fatal doses are on the order of micrograms and milligrams, respectively). Exotoxins are highly antigenic and are used to produce toxoids for vaccination. Most exotoxins are destroyed upon heating to 60°C, while endotoxins remain potent even after boiling.

64.C

Right-left orientation, as well as finger gnosis (naming) and calculation are functions of the dominant parietal lobe.

65.E; 66.B

Interferons (IFNs) are glycoproteins which inhibit viral growth, as well as the growth of bacteria, protozoa, and cancer cells. Alpha and beta IFN are induced by viruses, and gamma IFN is induced by antigens and increases the expression of class II MHC on antigen-presenting cells. Double-stranded RNA (a viral replication intermediate) and viruses are the strongest inducers of IFN; it is weakly induced by intracellular bacteria and endotoxin. The induction and action of

IFN are nonspecific. Lipoteichoic acid is found in the Gram positive cell wall, and ergosterol is found in fungal membranes.

67.B

Several bacteria produce toxins which ADP-ribosylate host targets. *C. diphtheria* exotoxin inactivates elongation factor 2 (EF-2) in this fashion (Diphtheria). Exotoxins from *E. coli, V. cholerae, B. pertussis*, and *B. cereus* all permanently stimulate adenylate cyclase by ADP-ribosylation. This results in an increase in intracellular cAMP and a consequent loss of chloride and water (diarrhea). The edema factor of *Bacillus anthracis* is similarly an adenylate cyclase. The exotoxin from *C. tetani* acts to block the release of the inhibitory neurotransmitter glycine through a different mechanism (Tetanus).

68.B

Stimulation of the medial hypothalamus of a cat results in rageful aggression (snarling, hissing, and attacking indiscriminately). Stimulation of the lateral hypothalamus results in predatory behavior (stalking and biting natural prey only).

69.D

The organisms most frequently isolated from blood cultures include *Pseudomonas aeruginosa*, *Escherichia coli* , *Klebsiella pneumoniae* as well as *Streptococcus pneumoniae. Shigella* tends to remains localized to the gastrointestinal mucosa.

70.C

Cholesterol is a neutral compound which alters the molecular packing of the cell membrane by inhibiting lateral movement of integral membrane components.

71.D

When $p < .05$, the results are statistically significant to the 95% confidence level, and the null hypothesis should be rejected.

72.E

Chi squared assesses the significance between proportions (frequencies). **T-test** analyzes the difference between means of two samples, while **ANOVA tests** differences between means of more than two samples. **Correlation tests** the mutual relation between two continuous variables, while regression analysis tests the relation between many measures.

73.C

Passive aggressive involves translating one's angry feelings into quiet defiances.

74.C

NSAIDs cause significant problems in the elderly and in patients with CHF, CRF and coagulopathy. They may cause significant GI bleeding, epigastric distress, nauseas and vomiting. They inhibit platelet agreggation and prolong the bleeding time. They may causes respiratory depression, and respiratory or metabolic acidosis. In children the use of salicylates has been correlated with Reye's syndrome (fulminant hepatitis with cerebral edema). They may exacerbate CRF by decreasing the glomerular flow. They also may increase the symptoms of CHF by retention of fluid. Pseudomembranous colitis is usually produced by proliferation of *C. difficile* after the administration of antibiotics.

75.D

The erthrocyte (RBC) utilizes glycolysis to produce ATP, pyruvate, and lactate from glucose. It can also produce carbon dioxide and NADPH using the hexose-monophosphate shunt. The RBC lacks mitochondria, and hence cannot use aerobic metabolism to produce acetyl CoA from pyruvate.

76.C

Eukaryotic mRNAs differ from prokaryotic mRNAs in that they have 5' methyl-guanine caps (which help align the ribosome with the start codon) and 3' poly(A) tails (which might protect the mRNA from degradation). The poly(A) tail is a post-transcriptional modification which is added by the enzyme poly(A) polymerase.

77.D

Schizophreniform disorder has all the diagnostic criteria of schizophrenia, but is of shorter duration than the six months required for a diagnosis of schizophrenia. Schizoaffective disorder has concurrent mood symptoms.

78.E

Reserpine is an alpha adrenergic blocker that has been implicated in the onset of depression, presumably due to its norepinepherine-depleting activity. Each of the other modalities has been shown to be of value in treating depression.

79.C

Anhedonia is seen in a variety of clinical settings. The other definitions describe agoraphobia (A), abulia (B), apraxia or ataxia (D), and aphasia (E).

80.A

Antipsychotic medications act by blocking dopamine (D2) receptors. Common side effects of these medications include sedation (uncommon with clozapine and haloperidol), orthostatic hypotension (uncommon with haloperidol), extrapyramidal symptoms (EPS; uncommon with thioridazine and clozapine), and anticholinergic effects (uncommon with haloperidol).

81.E

Transduction may be generalized (when a fragmented piece of DNA is incorporated into the viral particle during assembly), or specialized (when an integrated virus is excised and leaves the cell). Other means to transfer DNA between cells include **conjugation** (between two bacteria connected by pili) and **transformation** (uptake of naked DNA). **Recombination** (integration into the bacterial chromosome) is a process which may occur after new DNA has entered the cell.

82.C

There are 64 possible tRNAs (61 of which code for amino acids) and 20 standard amino acids. Because the third codon position is flexible in its base-pairing affinity, («wobble»), a single tRNA species can bind to multiple codons. Hence, the genetic code is degenerate. The statement in the alternative (a) is true but not germane to the question. Introns are removed prior to translation. Noncoding DNA is generally not transcribed.

83.B

An antisense RNA molecule can base pair with the mRNA of a targeted gene and thus prevent protein expression. A palindromic sequence reads the same backward and forward.

84.E

One-word speech and standing are normal developmental milestones for one year. Rolling over, sitting, and walking typically begin at 5, 7, and 15 months respectively.

85.B

Wave types, from fastest to slowest, are beta, alpha, theta, and delta. Beta occurs during attentiveness, alpha during relaxation, and delta in deep sleep. Focal delta and theta waves may indicate pathology.

86.D

The mini-mental state test is a standardized screening tool with a maximum score of 30. It tests orientation, registration and recall, attention and calculation, and language skills (such as reading, writing, copying, and following commands). Abstract reasoning may be tested separately, for example by asking a subject to interpret a metaphor.

87.C; 88.D

The figure shows a typical seminoma with large and round-to-polyhedral cells (seminoma cells) with a distinct cell membrane, and a large, central hyperchromatic nucleus with one or two prominent nucleoli. Several lymphocytes are also present in 80% of the patients. Seminoma is the most common type of germinal tumor (30%). They usually occur in the fourth decade. Three variants are described: typical (85%), anaplastic (5 - 10%), and spermatocytic (4 -6 %). It is most frequent between the ages 25-55 years and is not found before puberty. It is exquisitely sensitive to radiation therapy. Even in more advanced stages, chemotherapy is curative in 90% of the cases.

89.C

Interferons are produced by animal cells after viral infection. They act nonspecifically to block viral protein translation.

90.A

Tumor necrosis factor α reduces fatty acid utilization by inhibiting lipoprotein lipase, a cell-surface enzyme which hydrolyzes triacylglycerols in lipoproteins in adipose tissue.

USMLE step 1

BASIC MEDICAL SCIENCES

BOOK F TEST 6

ANSWERS

1.A

H. influenza is the leading cause of meningitis in children. It causes upper respiratory infections and sepsis in children. In adults causes pneumonia, particularly in smokers and COPD with chronic bronchitis. It is a gram negative rod (coccobacillus) with a polysaccharide capsule. Growth requires factor X and factor V in agar chocolate. The treatment of choice in meningitis is ceftriazone. In COPD and bronchitis, any second o third generation cephalosporins, ampicillin, chloramphenicol, and bactrim are effective.

2.C

Lactose consists of α galactose and α glucose molecule in α ß(1,4) linkage. Branch points in glycogen occur about every 15 glucose molecules and are linked by α (1,6) bonds. In starch, amylopectin is branched, and amylose contains only α (1,4) bonds.

3.E

Carbohydrates are only absorbed in monosaccharide form. ß-Galactosidase (lactase) is deficient in 5-15% of white American adults and up to 80% of Asian- and African-American adults. Unabsorbed lactose remains osmotically active in the intestinal lumen and often leads to diarrhea. Deficiencies in the enzymes oligo-1,6-glucosidase (isomaltase), α-glucosidase (maltase), ß-glucosidase, and trehalase which is specific for α(1,1) glucose bonds are much less common.

4.A

S_3 and S_4 (produced respectively by early passive and late contractile ventricular filling) are normally very quiet. A loud S_3/S_4 gallop rhythm typically results from increased resistance to filling due to decreased compliance (in hypertensive disease or post-myocardial infarction), or increased stroke volume in high-output states. It is most frequent in older persons.

5.A

The sharp «thud» is due to turbulent flow of blood as the cuff pressure decreases to equal the systolic blood pressure. The diastolic measurement is generally accepted as the pressure at which turbulent flow ceases and no sound is heard. An auscultatory gap is a period of silence between the systolic and diastolic pressures.

6.D; 7.A

The primary derangement in Parkinson's disease is the atrophy of the dopamine-producing substantia nigra. L-dopa is often used as replacement therapy. However, L-dopa is subject to inactivation via peripheral decarboxylation. Carbidopa is a useful adjunct in that it inhibits the peripheral decarboxylation of L-dopa, thereby making it possible to decrease the required dose of L-dopa.

8.E

Hexokinase (HK) catalyzes the first reaction of glycolysis: the ATP-dependent phosphorylation of glucose at C-6. HK exists as four isozymes. Isozymes I-III are widely distributed, while HK IV (glucokinase, GK) is found only in the liver. GK is highly specific for glucose and has a higher K_M than HK (10 mM vs. 0.1 mM), making it more responsive to small changes in blood glucose levels. HK operates near V_{max} at normal substrate concentrations.

9.B

Phosphofructokinase (PFK) converts fructose-6-phosphate to fructose-1,6-bisphosphate (F-1,6-BP). Like hexokinase, PFK is dependent upon ATP. An allosteric enzyme, PFK is a primary site for regulation of glycolysis; it is activated by AMP, ADP, F-1,6-BP, and F-2,6-BP and is inhibited by citrate and ATP. PK and PGK catalyze subsequent glycolytic reactions which produce ATP.

10.C

The pulsed secretion of GnRH, which prior to menstruation is inhibited by progesterone, triggers a surge of LH, which triggers ovulation. High estrogen levels at midcycle also facilitate ovulation.

11.E

The following table describes the differences between the types of muscle fibers.

Characteristic	Type I (red)	Type IIA **(red)**	Type IIB **(white)**
Type	slow, oxidative	fast, oxidat.	fast, glycolytic
Diameter	moderate	small	large
Innervation	small nerves	large	large
SR pumping capacacity	moderate	high	high
Myosin isozyme	slow	fast	fast
Contractions	slow, prolonged	rapid, powerful	rapid, powerful

12.A; 13.C; 14.D

Propantheline is a muscarinic receptor antagonist which promotes mucosal healing by blocking the vagus nerve. **Cimetidine** competitively block the H2 histamine receptor, thus decreasing acid secretion and promoting healing of the ulcer. **Omeprazole** inhibits the gastric H+/-K+-ATPase, a membrane-bound proton pump. It is effective in the management of gastric acid hypersecretion. **Misoprostol** causes ulcer healing and pain relief in both gastric and duodenal ulcer. It is an analog of prostaglandin E1, with antisecretory and cytoprotective properties. It is effective in the reducing mucosal damage resulting from the chronic administration of NSAIDs.

15.A

IL-2 and gamma IFN both stimulate CMI, while IL-4 is a B cell growth factor. Thus, the measles virus weakens CMI and delayed-type hypersensitivity, the most effective branch of immunity for handling viruses. Immunoglobulin levels are usually normal.

16.B

A prototypical polypeptide growth factor receptor, the FGFR is composed of an extracellular ligand-binding domain that contains three immunoglobulin-like domains, a single transmembrane domain, and a cytoplasmic domain that contains protein kinase activity. FGFR activation leads to receptor autophosphorylation, dimerization, internalization, and phosphorylation of specific target substrates, which triggers a cascade leading to various biological responses.

17.A

Monosaccharides are usually transferred to growing sugar polymers by first being placed in a higher energy form through conjugation to uridine diphosphate (UDP). UDP is released after the glycosidic linkage is formed. For example, lactose is synthesized by adding UDP-galactose to glucose in a reaction catalyzed by glu-UDP galactosyl transferase.

18.B

Average adult values for heart rate and blood pressure are 72 beats/min and 120/80 mmHg. For infants, the expected range is 120-170 for heart rate and 60-96 mmHg systolic and 30-62 mmHg diastolic.

19.D

Halothane is converted to trifluoroacetic acid, which is especially toxic to the liver. The other drugs derive some therapeutic efficacy from their metabolites. **Heroin** and codeine are both converted to morphine. **Diazepam** is converted to oxazepam, and prednisone is inactive until converted to prednisolone.

20.D; 21.C

Zollinger-Ellison syndrome is an islet cell tumor consisting of G cells, which secrete gastrin, a potent secretogogue for acid in the stomach. Among islet cell tumors pancreatic gastrinoma is second in frequency only to insulinomas. It is common between the ages of 30 and 50 years. In 15% of the cases the tumor may arise from from duodenal tissue. **Glucagonomas** or alpha cell tumors are associated with a syndrome consisting in mild diabetes, anemia, venous thrombosis, erythematous necrotizing, migratory rash, and severe infections.

22.E; 23.A

Proproxyphene is a derivative of methadone used as an analgesic to relieve mild to moderate pain. **Phenobarbital** is an antiepileptic drug useful in elemental partial seizures. It is a sedative-hypnotic and anticonvulsant. **Dextroamphetamine** is an CNS stimulant similar to cocaine. It is also a peripheral vasopressor. The mechanism by which it controls the symptoms of attention deficit disorder with hyperactivity in children is not well established. **Diazepam** is a benzodiazepine which has a potent anxiolytic effect. It is also used as a sedative, anticonvulsivant and muscle relaxant. **Chloropromazine** is a neuroleptic drug useful in the treatment of psychotic symptoms.

24.C

Gluconeogenesis (GNG) requires bypass reactions to replace irreversible glycolysis enzymes. Pyruvate kinase is bypassed by two enzymes in GNG (via an oxaloacetate intermediate): pyruvate carboxylase and phophoenolpyruvate carboxykinase (PEPCK). Phosphofructokinase is replaced by fructose bisphosphatase, and hexokinase is bypassed by glucose-6-phosphatase

25.B; 26.A; 27.D; 28.E

The citric acid cycle occurs in the mitochondrial matrix and functions to produce carbon dioxide and reduced electron carriers for the respiratory chain. In the diagram, citrate synthase (1) catalyzes the condensation of acetyl CoA (from glycolysis) and oxaloacetate (OAA; E) to form citrate, which is isomerized by aconitase (2). Isocitrate dehydrogenase (3) generates α-ketoglutarate (aKG- A). Next, α KG dehydrogenase (4) forms succinyl-CoA (B) from α KG. Succinyl-CoA synthetase (5) catalyzes the formation of succinate (C) from succinyl-CoA, and the consequent substrate-level phosphorylation of GDP to GTP. Succinate dehydrogenase (6) produces fumarate and reduces FAD to $FADH_2$. Fumarase (7) catalyzes the hydration of the fumarate double-bond to form malate (D); Malate dehydrogenase (8) converts malate to OAA (E); this highly endergonic reaction (ΔGo' = +29.7) proceeds because citrate synthase keeps intramitochondrial OAA levels very low. Three molecules of NADH are produced by each turn of the cycle, one each at steps 3, 4, and 8.

29.A; 30.C

Normally, senescent erythrocytes are degraded in the spleen, releasing heme, which is oxygenated to biliverdin and then reduced to bilirubin (BR). In the bloodstream, BR is transported bound to albumin. In the liver, BR is conjugated with two glucuronic acid residues, and the hydrophilic BR-diglucuronide enters the bile. Intestinal bacterial hydrolases remove the glucuronide groups, and free BR is reduced to urobilinogen, which is oxidized to colored products (urobilins) and expelled in the feces. In hemolytic jaundice («C»), BR levels exceed the body's metabolic and excretory capabilities. In obstructive jaundice («A»), a blockade at a biliary duct prevents conjugated BR from entering the intestine. In hepatocellular jaundice («E»), due to infectious hepatitis or cirrhosis, the liver's conjugation capacity is decreased.

31.A

Dronabinol, commonly known as Δ9 THC, is one of the major active substances in marijuana. It is currently approved for lessening the nausea and vomiting associated with cancer chemotherapy, and is under investigation as an appetite stimulant for AIDS patients. Dronabinol has complex effects upon the central nervous system and a high potential for abuse and dependence. It potentiates the effects of sympathomimetics, anticholinergic and tricyclic drugs. Concomitant phenothiazines may reduce toxicities.

32.C, 33.A, 34.E

In maple syrup urine disease, the enzyme complex which catabolizes branched-chain amino acids (leu, ile, and val) is defective. Alpha-ketoacid intermediates (which have a characteristic odor) accumulate in the urine. **Homocystinuria**, characterized by mental retardation and dislocation of the optic lens, results from a deficiency in cystathionine synthase. **Homocystine** (an oxidation product from a normally inactive pathway) accumulates in the urine. **CF**, the most common fatal autosomal recessive disorder among white children, has a carrier frequency of about 1 in 22. Mutations in the CF transmembrane conductance regulator (CFTM) render it unresponsive to cAMP, which decreases the secretion of chloride and associated fluid. The resultant thick mucus obstructs the lumina of airways, pancreatic and biliary ducts, and the fetal intestine. PKU results from a heterogeneous group of autosomal recessive mutations in phenylalanine hydroxylase, the enzyme that converts phe to tyr. Phe accumulates in body fluids, damaging the developing central nervous system. Alternative metabolites (such as phenylpyruvic acid) are excreted in the urine. Lesch-Nyhan syndrome is an X-linked absence of hypoxanthine guanine phosphoribosyltransferase (HPRT), which converts hypoxanthine to IMP and guanine to GMP. The lack of feedback inhibition increases de novo purine synthesis. Symptoms include hyperuricemia, choreoathetosis, spasticity, mental retardation, and self-mutilation.

35.A

Oxaloacetate (OAA) is synthesized in the mitochondria by pyruvate carboxykinase; it is converted to aspartate, for which there is a specific carrier. The aspartate is then transaminated back to OAA in the cytoplasm, where PEPCK and the other enzymes of gluconeogenesis are located. OAA is also produced from malate in a reaction which generates NADH.

36.A

The sympathetic system is involved in «fight or flight» responses. It uses epinephrine and norepinephrine as its primary neurotransmitters. Functions include pupillary and bronchial dilation, increased heart rate and contractility, and decreased digestive processes.

37.D

DNA moves in an electric field on the basis of it size and charge; smaller fragments will move faster and thus farther compared to larger fragments. In the figure, the plasmid is moving slower in lane B compared to lane A; this could be explained by the insertion of another DNA sequence (which would make the plasmid larger and slower). Supercoiled DNA is more compact and thus moves faster. A fragmented plasmid would appear as multiple smaller bands. Diluting the sample would simply weaken the intensity of the band.

38.D

DNA is negatively charged, primarily by virtue of the acidic phosphate groups in the backbone. Recalling that «opposites attract,» DNA will move toward the positive pole, which is the cathode.

39.D

Sphingosine is a long-chain amino alcohol consisting of palmitate and serine. A **cerebroside** is a ceramide (sphingosine plus a fatty acid) plus a sugar group (such as galactose or glucosamine). A **ganglioside** is a ceramide plus multiple sugar groups.

40.C

The human erythrocyte is a classic model of membrane structure. By weight, it consists of 49% protein, 43% lipid, and 8% carbohydrate. Of the lipid fraction, about 25% is cholesterol. Other lipid components include glycerophospholipids such as phoshatidylcholine (19%) and phosphatidylethanolamine (18%); sphingomyelin (17.5%), and various glycolipids (10%).

41.E; 42.D

Damaged myocardial cells release characteristic intracellular enzymes into the serum. LDH consists of four subunits of two types, H (heart) and M (skeletal muscle). LDH_1 (HHHH) and LDH_2 (HHHM) begin to increase 24-48 h after an MI, peak around 96 h, and gradually fall over two weeks, making LDH a good long-term indicator. CK exists as three isozymes: brain (BB), skeletal muscle (MM), and cardiac (MB). After an MI, CK(MB) levels rise faster (4-24 h) and return to normal earlier (48-72 h) compared to LDH. AST (formerly known as SGOT) is normally expressed in both heart and liver tissue, while ALT (formerly SGPT) predominates in liver, a distribution which can aid in diagnosis. AST and ALT are beginning to fall out of favor, because they rise and fall at times intermediate to LDH and CK, and have less tissue specificity. Troponins T and I are newer indicators which are highly sensitive, cardiospecific, and rise rapidly (2-4 h) following MI. These advantages may make troponins the markers of choice in the future.

43.B; 44.E; 45.A

Procainamide is a Group 1A cardiac antiarrhythmic drug chemically related to the local anesthetic procaine. It inhibits automaticity and reduces myocardial excitability and conduction velocity.

Hydralazine lowers blood pressure in hypertensive individuals by peripheral vasodilatation through a direct relaxation of vascular smooth muscle. Hydralazine alters cellular calcium metabolism but has not been shown to be selective for adrenergic receptors. Both drugs may produce a multisystem lupus-like syndrome of arthralgia, myalgia, pleural effusion, glomerulonephritis, etc. **Verapamil** is a calcium channel blocker useful in the treatment of supraventricular tachyarrhythmias. **Nitrates** (nitroglycerin) are useful as an anti-angina medication.

46.C

Digoxin Immune Fab (Digibind) consists of specific antidigoxin antibodies which bind digoxin. The resulting complexes accumulate in the blood and are excreted by the kidney. It is indicated for potentially life-threatening digoxin overdose.

47.C

Pyruvate represents a metabolic crossroads. It can complete glycolysis aerobically (conversion to acetyl CoA by pyruvate dehydrogenase) or anaerobically (conversion to lactate by lactate dehydrogenase), or it can lead to gluconeogenesis (conversion to oxaloacetate by pyruvate carboxylase). In yeast, pyruvate is also decarboxylated to acetaldehyde, which is converted to ethanol by alcohol dehydrogenase.

48.C; 49.A

Oligonucleotide mutagenesis is performed by constructing a DNA sequence which is nearly complementary to a target DNA sequence. By hybridizing these sequences and extending the synthetic primer, the newly polymerized DNA molecule will differ from the parent at the chosen site. Linker scanning mutagenesis involves the generation of a random set of deletion mutants. DNase I protection mapping (footprinting) can identify protein-DNA binding sites, as unbound DNA is enzymatically fragmented. A mobility shift assay is a method to detect DNA binding proteins in crude protein extracts. ELISA offers a way to quantify antigens or antibodies.

50.D

The right renal vein (along with the duodenum and the uncinate process of the pancreas) lies in the acute angle between the superior mesenteric artery and the aorta.

51.C

The small cardiac vein parallels the marginal branch of the RCA. The anterior veins usually arise from the RCA proper. The great and middle cardiac veins travel with the left anterior descending and right posterior interventricular branches respectively. Thesbian veins drain the myocardium directly to the heart chambers.

52.A

The inferior epigastric vein empties into the external iliac vein. Direct inguinal hernias are medial to and indirect hernias are lateral to the inferior epigastic vein.

53.B

General anesthetics are hydrophobic compounds which appear to act via membrane expansion rather than receptor binding. Blood : gas solubility (S) is related to equilibration rate. Agents with a high S (eg., halothane) equilibrate slowly and are respiration limited. Agents with a low S (eg., nitrous oxide) equilibrate rapidly and are limited by cardiac output. MAC (minimal alveolar concentration) is a measure of potency.

54.E

Amrinone is a vasodilator with cardiac stimulant properties. **Dipyridamole** is a phosphodiesterase inhibitor, and caffeine is a methylxanthine. **Dobutamine** is a beta-1 agonist. **Bretylium** is a class III antiarrhythmic agent which prolongs the refractory period and delays repolarization of myocardium.

55.C, 56.A

Tamoxifen is an estrogen antagonist which is used in the therapy of estrogen-receptor positive breast cancer. **Clomiphene** may induce ovulation in anovulatory women, apparently through an increased output of pituitary gonadotropins. Multiple pregnancies occur in up to 10% of conceptions. **Ethinyl estradiol** and mestranol are both synthetic estrogens, and norethindrone is a progestin.

57.D

The **Cori cycle** functions to provide glucose to extrahepatic tissue (such as contracting muscle) during anaerobic glycolysis. Lactate is transported to the liver, where it is converted to pyruvate and then glucose, which is transported back to muscle. The overall process is energy-consuming.

58.B

The enzymes involved in glycogen synthesis and degradation are regulated by covalent modification. Glycogen synthetase b (inactive) is activated by protein phosphatase I. The resulting glycogen synthetase a (active) is inactivated by the addition of a phosphate group, catalyzed by various kinases, such as glycogen synthase kinase-3. In contrast, phosphorylase which catalyzes glycogen breakdown is active («a») when phosphorylated and inactive («b») when dephosphorylated.

59.D

Glycogen storage diseases (GSD) result from inactivation of any of several enzymes of glycogen metabolism and can have severe clinical consequences. Types Ia and Ib GSD involve deficiencies of glucose-6-phosphatase (G6Pase) and G6Pase translocase, respectively. Type II GSD involves a deficiency in a (1->4) glucosidase. Muscle glycogen phosphorylase is deficient in type V GSD. Glycogen structure is normal in each of the above diseases. In contrast, glycogen in type III GSD, in which debranching enzyme is deficient, shows short outer chains, while glycogen in type IV GSD (in which branching enzyme is deficient) shows abnormally long unbranched chains.

60.A

Fatty acids are long chain hydrocarbons (10-22 carbons) with terminal carboxyl groups. Fatty acids of intermediate chain length and zero to two double bonds are most commonly found in biological lipids. Common examples include myristic acid (14 carbons, 0 double bonds), palmitic acid (16:0), stearic acid (16:0), palmitoleic acid (16:1), oleic acid (18:1), linoleic acid (18:2), linolenic acid (18:3), and arachidonic acid (20:4). Melting points of fatty acids tend to decrease with increasing degree of unsaturation.

61.A

Chromatography is used to isolate and purify biomolecules. In gel filtration chromatography, the soluble (mobile) sample interacts with a stationary phase as it is passed through a column containing inert particles of a fixed pore size. Small molecules are eluted more rapidly than large molecules. The other chromatographic methods listed rely on other characteristics, such as charge and biological interaction.

62.C

If protein X is made in this cell type, it will be specified by a genomic and mRNA sequence. Using *in situ* hybridization, a radiolabelled probe complementary to the gene or mRNA of interest could be constructed. Binding the probe to a cellular library and autoradiography would be sufficient to show that the protein is synthesized in the cell it is located in. Fluorescent monoclonal antibodies and western blotting would not be able to distinguish synthesized from stored protein.

63.A

To subclone the gene from the first plasmid to the second, restriction enzymes must be chosen such that the gene remains intact and cohesive ends will be present on the recipient plasmid. Although enzymes B and D most closely delimit the gene, there is no restriction site for B on the recipient plasmid, which would make a successful ligation more complicated Thus, enzyme A is a better choice.

64.C

The correct band contains the 1.2 kB gene (plus a small extra 5' sequence) plus the 7.0 kB pGEM plasmid (minus the small sequence between restriction sites A and D). The 7.6 band is closest to the expected length. The other bands are original plasmids, fragments, or other recombinant molecules.

65.B

The ulnar nerve arises from the medial cord of the brachial plexus and passes behind the medial epicondyle at the elbow, where it is vulnerable to injury. It provides sensory innervation to the medial side of the hand, including fifth and medial half of the fourth fingers.

66.D

Of the muscles listed, the splenius muscles are located most superficially in the back. Deep to these are the erector spinalis group consisting of the spinalis, iliocostalis, and longissimus. Deeper still is the transversospinalis group, consisting of the rotatores, multifidus, and semispinalis. All of these muscles are involved in extension and/or rotation of the back.

67.C

The posterior cricoarytenoid muscle facillitates breathing by opening the glottis. The lateral cricoarytenoids and the transverse thyroarytenoids close the glottis. The thyroarytenoids close the glottis and decrease tension on the vocal cords. The cricothyroid muscle increases tension on the vocal cords.

68.A

Daunorubicin inhibits DNA synthesis; it is antimitotic and cytotoxic. It is especially useful in the treatment of some forms of leukemia. Bone marrow depression and cardiac toxicity are among the potential adverse effects.

69.E; 70.B; 71.C

Self-explanatory.

72.B

The anabolic pentose phosphate pathway utilizes glucose-6-phosphate to generate NADPH, which is needed for fatty acid and steroid biosynthesis. The pathway also produces ribose-5-phosphate, a nucleotide building block. ATP is not produced directly, but can be made by diverting intermediates to the TCA cycle.

73.B

Facilitated transport is a saturable process; the rate of transport approaches a maximum when all facilitators are occupied. Carrier-facilitators are more sensitive to decreases in membrane fluidity (as occurs when the temperature is lowered below the fluid-gel transition temperature) than are pore-facilitators. Active transport can occur against a concentration gradient.

74.A

Ketogenic amino acids are converted to acetyl CoA or acetoacetate, precursors for ketone bodies. Trp, leu, and lys are strictly ketogenic. Amino acids which are both ketogenic and glucogenic include ile, phe, tyr, ala, gly, cys, ser, and thr. The other ten amino acids are strictly glucogenic.

75.E

Carbamoyl phosphate formed by the ATP-dependent reaction of ammonia and carbon dioxide, contributes the carbon and one nitrogen atom to urea. The other nitrogen atom comes from **aspartate** formed by the transamination of oxaloacetate with an amine group derived from glutamate. Four molecules of ATP are required to generate one molecule of urea.

76.C

Argininosuccinate synthetase, argininosuccinase, and arginase are present in the cytosol, while the other listed enzymes (including all the citric acid cycle enzymes) are present in the mitochondria.

77.E

Hormones produce a variety of cellular and molecular effects through diverse mechanisms. Options A through D are all plausible explanations for the scenario depicted in the question. However, ligand C and hormone P are not co-incubated in the given experimental design, and hence the hormone cannot directly induce a conformational change in the ligand.

78.A

Northern blotting is used to analyze the size and expression of specific mRNAs. RNA molecules are separated by size in a gel, transferred to nitrocellulose, and detected with a specific probe. Southern blotting is used to analyze DNA, and Western blotting is used to analyze proteins. HPLC and isoelectric focusing are also techniques used to analyze proteins.

79.C

The median nerve enters the wrist by passing through the carpal tunnel, behind the flexor retinaculum (which attaches laterally to the scaphoid and trapezium and medially to the pisiform and hamate bones.) Carpal tunnel syndrome results from compression of the nerve within this tunnel. Typically, symptoms consist of pain or tingling along the lateral three and one half fingers and weakness of the thenar muscles, which corresponds to the distribution of the median nerve. In question 5, option A describes a radial nerve palsy, and option D describes an ulnar nerve palsy.

80.C

The sternal angle (the joint between the manubrium

and body of the sternum) is an important landmark in the anterior chest. It articulates with the second rib and overlies T2.

81.C

Apoptosis (programmed cell death) of the cells at the junction between the embryonic fingers is necessary for the separation of the fingers.

82.C

On a dry weight basis, proteins and carbohydrates store 4 kcal/g, and fats store 9 kcal/g. In this case, 4(5+8) + 9(6) = 106 kcal.

83.B

Lipoprotein lipase, located at the adipocyte plasma membrane, allows free fatty acids to be absorbed. Hormone-sensitive lipase (triacylglycerol lipase) mediates lipolysis; it is activated by glucagon and epinephrine and inhibited by insulin. Insulin helps to clear the blood of fatty acids and glucose after meals.

84.A

During early starvation, gluconeogenesis in the liver maintains glucose («B») levels, while lipolysis from adipose tissue modestly increases serum fatty acids («C»). Ketone bodies («A»), such as acetoacetate and ß-hydroxybutyrate, are produced from acetyl-CoA and are utilized for energy by many tissues. During fasting, insulin levels would be expected to decrease and glucagon levels would be expected to increase. Glycogen is not released into the circulation.

85.D

Fatty acids are conjugated to coenzyme A and then transported into the mitochondrial matrix through a carnitine carrier. ß-oxidation involves a cycle of dehydrogenation, hydration, dehydrogenation, and thiolytic cleavage to yield acetyl CoA and a fatty acyl CoA of length (n-2). The substrate for the last cycle of an odd-chain acyl-CoA is a five carbon molecule, which is cleaved to form acetyl CoA and propionyl-CoA. Propionyl CoA is carboxylated to form methylmalonyl-CoA, which is converted to succinyl CoA by an enzyme (methylmalonyl CoA mutase) requiring vitamin B_{12}.

86.E

The methyl group on the ß-carbon of phytanic acid (derived from phytol, a constituent of chlorophyll) prevents ß-oxidation of this compound. An additional pathway involving alpha-oxidation occurs in peroxisomes; ß-oxidation subsequently occurs on the rest of the molecule. Alpha-oxidation is defective in patients with Refsum's disease. Chlorophyll (in green vegetables and meat from herbivores) must be avoided. Medium-chain acyl dehydrogenase (MCAD) deficiency is a more common genetic defect.

87.D

The tendons of the peroneus longus and brevis pass behind the lateral malleolus. The peroneus tertius tendon passes anterior to the lateral malleolus. The tendons of the tibialis posterior, flexor hallucis longus, and flexor digitorum longus pass behind the medial malleolus.

88.B

The unpaired anterior spinal artery travels in the anterior spinal sulcus and supplies the anterior 2/3 of the spinal cord. The paired posterior spinal arteries travel near the spinal nerve roots and supply the posterior 1/3 of the spinal cord. The spinal cord travels in the vertebral foramen, and the vertebral arteries travel in the transverse foraminae.

89.E

The ascending pharyngeal and superior thyroid arteries both originate proximal to the lingual artery. The facial, occipital, posterior auricular, superficial temporal, and maxillary arteries all branch off the external carotid artery distal to the lingual artery and hence would be compromised.

90.E

Sphingolipidoses (lipid storage diseases) are a group of congenital disorders characterized by lysosomal accumulation of the substrate for a deficient enzyme. Gaucher's disease involves a deficiency of ß-galactosidase. Normally, sphingolipids are metabolized to ceramide, which is degraded into sphingosine and fatty acid by ceramidase (which is deficient in Farber's lipogranulomatosis).